WHAT ABOUT IMMUNIZATIONS?
Exposing the Vaccine Philosophy

A parents' guide to the vaccination decision

Cynthia Cournoyer

Third edition © 1986;   fourth edition © 1987 *(second printing © 1988, third printing, revised © 1989, fourth printing © 1990)*;   fifth edition © 1991

ISBN: 0-9612188-4-3

printed on recycled paper

Cover Design:
    Zona Designs, Grants Pass, Oregon
    Copy Rite, Canby, Oregon
    Bulletin Printing, Grants Pass, Oregon

Typesetting:
    Litho-Logic Designs, Grants Pass, Oregon

Published by:
    Nelson's Books
    P.O. Box 2302
    Santa Cruz, CA 95063

What About Immunizations?

This book is dedicated to all children who have suffered as a result of vaccines. We pray their loss will someday wake up the world for the benefit of countless children everywhere.

ACKNOWLEDGMENTS

Special thanks to my husband who never stops encouraging me. Special thanks to my three children for giving me a reason to care and for sharing me with the typewriter. Special thanks to the special friends who "brought out the best in me" and trusted that I would come through. You all helped make this book possible.

Thanks also to everyone who sent articles, helped research, and provided feedback. Thanks to those other organizations and publications who continue to provide parents with the information they need to make a truly informed decision about vaccines.

**If We Rely On Knowledge
Without Common Sense
To Guide Us,
We Are Vulnerable
To Illusion**

Contents

PREFACE

This book offers a contrast to every-day information. It is especially for those searching parents who have suffered an onslaught of "facts" that go contrary to their original doubt. Parents are faced with a mountain of printed material that "sells" childhood vaccines* as if there was never any controversy. Virtually any month of the year, there is a parent-type magazine running an article explaining how wonderful and important vaccines are to the total health care of a child.

The majority of children's doctors and health departments "inform" the parents with partial facts or none, and usually add fear and pressure if too many questions are asked. In addition, co-workers, sisters, mothers, grannies, in-laws, back-fence neighbors and life-long friends chatter in parents' ears about how it is a duty to see that their child is "protected" from "preventable" diseases.

A vaccine is designed to give a person the disease in a "milder" form, in hopes that the body will "remember" how to fight if off. One begins to doubt something that makes a child sick could make a child better.

Realizing there are no easy answers when it comes to vaccines,

---

*The words, "vaccine" or "vaccination" and "immunization" are commonly used interchangeably. Because a person can be *naturally* immune, a definite distinction must be made. Vaccines are manufactured and so can be considered *artificial* when it comes to defining true immunity. Therefore, the word "vaccines" will be consistently used throughout this book where others might refer to childhood "immunizations."

parents are motivated to find confirmation of their common sense beliefs. Purely driven with the desire to do what's best for their children, parents soon learn that making a decision can be very emotional.

After nine years of tracking many parents as they made a difficult decision whether to vaccinate their child, this book has evolved into a helpful examination of these psychological and emotional aspects of vaccine decision-making. It does not offer medical advice, as the author is not a physician, rather the parents' peer... a "good friend" when all seems confusing and little makes sense. There is enough information in this book to give a reader the confidence to stand up to any pro-vaccine argument, no matter how sophisticated.

Making a decision, one way or the other, does not imply a parent has taken the final step. Various degrees of confidence, alternating with self-doubt, will have constant influence. Parents may find themselves refining their decisions regarding childhood vaccines. Careful thought has gone into the development of this book, considering the journey that a parent is likely to make. As opinions and convictions are formed, and understanding takes hold, this book stands as a permanent guide with which parents may periodically refer.

What About Immunizations? can help decode the language of the vaccine philosophers. Exposing the "vaccine philosophy" puts into perspective the available choices, so a parent can make an informed decision. Almost as important as an informed decision is the parents' ability to be comfortable with that decision. Because ultimately, when all is said and done, the parents and the child must live with it for the rest of their lives.

Part I

Vaccinating — An Overview

THE VACCINE PHILOSOPHY *

"Philosophy and science differ in many respects. For example, science has attained definite and tested knowledge of many matters and has thus resolved disagreement about those matters. Philosophy has not. As a result, controversy has always been characteristic of philosophy."

The World Book Encyclopedia, 1988

The vaccine philosophy leads to the conclusion that vaccines are safe and effective and that the benefits outweigh the risks. The controversy rises out of continuing evidence contrary to these traditionally-held beliefs.

Vaccination is based on questionable theories, but through

* The author coined the term, "vaccine philosophy." It is defined here and used throughout this book.

1

cultural conditioning, it is almost unanimously accepted. The bottom line is people *want* to believe vaccines work and they will find "evidence" to support these beliefs. But, for every "fact" supporting these beliefs, there is another fact that counters it. Therefore, one is left alone in a "sea of facts" to decide which he *chooses* to believe. A person will either believe in vaccination theories or he will not. Those who concur with the traditional thoughts on vaccines are said to believe in the "vaccine philosophy."

A new vaccine must first be *assumed* safe and effective until it is proven otherwise sometime in the future. So, people hang on to that assumption and it becomes commonly accepted, regardless of suggestions to the contrary.

Vaccination is not a pure basic science. Once a vaccine has been approved for general use, it is no longer ethical to withhold a vaccine and give a placebo in its place in order to compare results in two groups of the population.[1] A legitimate control group does not exist. "Scientists" will use the general population as their "control group" *even though the general population is 90% vaccinated.* After using "X" vaccine, they "find no more occurrence of encephalitis (for example) than would be expected to occur in the general population."

Too many variables go unaccounted. Too many questions go unanswered. For instance, no study has ever compared developmental or cognitive function in vaccinated and unvaccinated children. The control group is also vaccinated. One cannot compare vaccinated children with other vaccinated children and hope to arrive at a valid estimate of the percentage that experience side effects, whether immediate or delayed.

The more one understands the presuppositions that must be made in order to have faith in a vaccine, the more one doubts the entire philosophy behind vaccination. Yielding to the temptation of assuming too much simplicity is easy but leads to the faulty hypothesis: vaccines are safe and good. This is the presupposition of almost every vaccine "study." The only unanswered questions would be, *"how* safe and *how* good?" This never allows for the consideration that the opposite hypothesis (that vaccines are inherently dangerous) may be much more scientific and provide sturdier ground on which to build medical theories.

While stubbornly sticking to a faulty hypothesis, studies will treat vaccine injury and vaccine ineffectiveness as an exception with reasons yet unknown. While assuming there is nothing wrong with vaccination, studies will go on to figure ways that could have prevented failure by simply changing *doses* or vaccine *procedures*.

Most studies are 100% focused on the benefits of vaccination to the point of outright denial of the risks. Negative findings are often ignored, manipulated or simply abandoned in order to prevent the risk of finding flaws in that original hypothesis. We do know that diseases vaccinated against, occur in both vaccinated and unvaccinated individuals, so without pure scientific evidence, the conclusion could just as easily be made that vaccines do not work.

It seems reasonable to question whether to give this vaccine or that vaccine, whether this one is safer than the next, etc. But choosing one vaccine over another does not escape the vaccine philosophy. It is still a belief without sound scientific principles.

Public awareness of negative aspects of vaccines is treated as a fringe element and never as a red flag signifying possible danger to America's children. Opposition to the vaccine philosophy is actively discouraged or squelched. The law is used to coerce if not force parents into succumbing to non-emergency medicine. The parents are injected with a sense of urgency that tugs on their emotions and pressures them into ignoring the possible dangers of vaccines because this has "already been deemed their best and only option."

The vaccine philosophy has invaded society to the extent that most do not question the procedure. Societal pressure and cultural conditioning bring most members of the community around to the status-quo. The mavericks pave the way for deeper probing. But, given both sides and a clear choice, a person will ultimately choose which best fits his outlook on life; he may make traditional choices, he may not.

We are comfortable in our belief system when it is constantly reinforced by the culture in which we live. Those who break away from this conditioning might consider vaccination ineffective and harmful and may look on those who vaccinate as being a member of an absurd culture that places their belief in the ceremony of vaccination.

It is natural to gather all kinds of information and examine and weigh each aspect. That is what most searching parents try to do with the vaccine issue. But without science squarely behind it, all that remains is belief. A person will ultimately act on what he *believes*. Some believe the vaccine philosophy, some do not.

THE GERM THEORY AND SCIENCE'S "LOST CHAPTER"

- **Bechamp or Pasteur?**

- **Soil for Disease**

- **Health and Vaccines**

- **What If?**

Bechamp or Pasteur?

> "The germ theory has suited man's ego quite well. Most of us prefer to believe that the illnesses we suffer are the result of external forces — just as we would rather blame bad luck for our failures." [2]

The willingness to accept vaccines so readily may have its roots back 130 years when two French scientists were researching what causes fermentation. The result eventually developed into the well accepted "germ theory." *Belief in vaccines* as a reasonable method of dealing with disease is based on the germ theory. *Fear of disease* is perpetuated by this germ theory. But if this germ theory were wrong, would we no longer be afraid of disease and find no need or desire for vaccines?

Pasteur (1822-1895) realized airborne microorganisms (later

known as bacteria) caused fermentation, then sought to explain his previous idea of spontaneous generation with the existence of "germs." He ignored those microorganisms *within* cells that cause fermentation and perform other important biological functions as well. He believed that the microorganisms were fixed entities and he divided them into different classes, claiming each group fermented one kind of food and another fermented another and so on. This eventually led to the theory that different bacteria cause different diseases. Pasteur's oversimplifications led to his theories becoming well promoted and easily accepted. [3]

Bechamp said that airborne organisms are simply microzymas or their evolutionary forms (bacteria) set free by decomposition of the plant or animal body in which they lived. These microzymas (Greek for small ferments), or cell granules, induce fermentation. Microzymas are constantly developing into bacteria. If tissue is healthy, they will function to support life and integrity of the cells. If the cells have been damaged they will produce morbid or diseased microzymas, which may evolve into pathogenic (disease-producing) bacteria. The microzyma has two functions: to build or to disintegrate tissue. Good health results from the balance of these two processes. [4]

Bechamp showed that bacteria function in whatever medium they find themselves, even changing their shapes and function in accordance with that medium. While looking into a microscope, Pasteur might have commented, "Ah, here is the bacteria that ferments beer and this is its shape." Bechamp might have said, "Here is a bacteria fermenting beer. In beer it takes on this shape." In other words, bacteria reflect the conditions in which they find themselves, rather than creating those conditions. [5]

> "Modern medicine, under the spell of the germ theory, tells us that for every disease there is a disease entity — individual bacteria shaped in a particular way — that causes a particular disease. Bechamp showed through innumerable experiments that not only is the germ we associate with a particular disease a *product* and *not the cause* of the disease, but also that what some researchers would call different species of

bacteria are really different stages of microzymian evolution into their bacterial forms. We might say that while Pasteur taught that germs cause disease, Bechamp taught that disease generates germs."[6]

There was a choice 130 years ago and we accepted the idea that germs attack at random and getting rid of the germ results in health. We should have chosen the idea that disease depends on the "soil" of the individual. This requires taking much more responsibility for one's individual health, therefore, it is not easily accepted.

Pasteur was a respected and influential man. Being a chemist and physicist, he knew very little about biology and life processes. His fear of infection, his belief in the "belligerence" of germs, and his powerful influence on his contemporaries, led men of science to be convinced of the threat of the microbe to man.[7]

A French physiologist, Claude Bernard (1813-1878) also disputed the validity of the Germ Theory, and maintained that the general condition of the body was the principal factor in disease. Bernard and Pasteur had many debates on the relative importance of the microbe and the internal environment.[8]

After numerous experiments, Pasteur was finally convinced that controllable physiological factors were basic in vulnerability to disease. He concluded that the presence of certain germs is not proof that they are the cause of a disease.[9]

Reversing his position and acknowledging that germs are not the primary cause of disease, Pasteur abandoned the Germ Theory. He is reported to have said on his deathbed: "Bernard was right. The seed is nothing, the soil is everything."[10]

> "But, like the third automobile, which was the proximate cause of the collision but proceeded on its way with impunity, Pasteur envisioned the truth in the 1880's, and abandoned the Germ Theory, leaving that early immature and erroneous theory to be developed, fostered, and perpetuated by others, the ultimate irony. The mischief, medical misunderstanding and error continue to this day, and the price is incalculable."
> [11]

Soil for Disease

We are constantly breathing in some 14,000 germs and bacteria per hour. If germs by themselves are the cause of all disease, we should be ill all the time. But it is the condition of the body that is the primary factor in whether a person will show signs of illness.

The frequency of inapparent infections out-number clinical illnesses by at least 100 times. Evidence for this is provided by the high proportion of people who have virus-neutralizing substances in their serum and the number who, during an epidemic excrete virus without becoming ill. [12]

In the winter and spring, approximately one person out of every four carries the meningitis bacteria in their nose. Most either develop mild flu-like symptoms or don't become ill at all. [13] Many people *carry* the microbes of influenza, tuberculosis, staphylococcus infections and many other illnesses, but this does not make them develop the disease. Every illness, no matter what the nature, is usually the consequence of a variety of causes, not just one, and no two people react to any one cause in the same way. [14] Often the afflicted and the non-afflicted are in the same household. [15] Furthermore, specific bacteria or germs are *not* found in every case of specific disease and specific bacteria are repeatedly found when the specific disease symptoms are not present. [16]

Injury to the inside of the body by stress and/or poor diet can reduce vitality and the body's ability to resist "germs" encountered in the environment. There must be some act of destruction for harmful bacteria to develop. A bruised or damaged fruit is far more susceptible to decay and rot than a perfect one. Healthy, undamaged human skin is extremely resistant to infection. Once gaining access to the inside of the body, the inner health of each cell is depended upon to resist the evolution of pathogenic bacteria.

Dead or decaying "food" must be present in order to culture bacteria. If the body is in a state of "decay," the microorganisms will be pathogenic. When the body is internally cleansed, pathogenic bacteria have nothing more to feed upon and the disease process reverses itself. [17] Disease symptoms such as fevers, mucous secretion, etc. have a cleansing effect. So it may not be as much a matter of "killing germs" but a matter of changing the "food" and starving the pathogenic bacteria.

A pneumococcus (pneumonia) bacteria can be reduced to a streptococcus back into a staphylococcus, simply by changing the growing medium in the lab.[18] The germ theory would theorize that each of those bacteria are separate entities and the only defense is to kill them. In these experiments they were not killed, only their food was changed, while allowing them to continue living. These experiments show conclusively that instead of bacteria determining how the environment will react (disease symptom) the environment actually determines which bacteria will grow.[19] Denied their exclusive type of food, moved from their natural habitat, and fed on other kinds of food, they quickly change into forms native to their new surroundings.

At the Mayo Biological Laboratories in 1910, Dr. Rosenow took bacterial strains from many different disease sources (peurperal sepsis, arthritis, tonsillitis and cow's milk) and put them into one culture of uniform media. Soon there was no difference between the germs; they all became of one class. He concluded there was no particularly fixed species of different germs and they all had the capacity to change their structure with the changes in their nutriments.[20] Many other experiments were carried out and in every instance, the germs, regardless of type, changed into other types when their food and environment were altered.

Germs seek their natural habitat (diseased tissues); they are not the cause of diseased tissue. Mosquitoes seek stagnant water but do not cause the pool to become stagnant.

A number of studies have shown that insects can detect subtle mineral imbalances in plants and destroy only those plants that are out of balance. Plants grown on organically mineralized and balanced soil do not attract pests nor do they get diseases as do plants grown on deficient and chemically fertilized soil. Satellite photographs have shown gigantic flights of locusts cover thousands of miles, ignoring healthy vegetation, then descend, destroying fields where the soil is worn out. Kirlian photography and other energy measuring devices have shown that the cells of every life form, plant, animal, human, and microorganismic, emit radio signals and photons (light). A strong, healthy plant radiates wavelengths of a different frequency than that of an imbalanced, unhealthy one. Strong plants broadcast wavelengths that act as a protective screen against pests. [21]

Microorganisms are a product rather than a cause of disease. [22] If a microbe is to have any part in disease, it must find a suitable "soil" for it's activities. The condition of the host is of primary importance in the production of diseases. [23] Whether man lives in equilibrium with microbes or becomes their victim depends upon the circumstances under which he encounters them. [24] The human body is the "soil" that can determine health or disease.

Health and Vaccines

The body has its own methods of defense. If it is vital enough, it will resist all infections, if it isn't vital enough it won't. The vitality of the body cannot be changed for the better by introducing vaccines, which contain known toxic substances.

Clean diet, clean living, and a low stress environment have done more to eliminate and prevent diseases over thousands of years than any other form of intervention. If we rely on quick fixes and modern medical miracles to save us from bad diets, stressful and unclean living, then we get farther and farther from the true source of health: maintaining a healthy lifestyle, aiding the body's miraculous ability to resist diseases and to heal itself.

The World Health Organization has conceded that the best "vaccine" against common infectious diseases is an adequate diet. Despite this, they made it clear that they still intend to promote mass vaccination campaigns. In the seventeenth and eighteenth centuries, bad harvests were almost always followed by a large increase in the number of deaths from smallpox and fevers. [25] Are vaccines cheaper than good food? Do vaccines make for better political impressions?

Where society in general believes that there is an enemy (germs) that is unavoidable and attacks at random, most people choosing not to vaccinate are relieved to know that there is control over individual health. One way in which we help our immune system is to control what goes into the body. The relationship between imbalance and toxicity can be demonstrated with nutrition. Refined white sugar and flour produce toxic metabolites such as pyruvic acid and abnormal sugars containing five carbon atoms which interfere with cell respiration and eventually the function of a part of the body. This begins the degenerative disease process. The United States leads the world in the incidence of degenerative disease *and* the consumption of refined food. Coincidence? In 1979 we were almost 40th place in national health. [26]

Avoiding germs is *not* the single factor in maintaining health. As with diet, there are other factors under our control. Emotional stress is associated with immune system dysfunction, lowered resistance and more severe forms of infection. [27] According to Norman Shealy, M.D., joy increases the strength of the immune system and sadness or depression decreases the strength of the immune system. Negative emotions trigger the release of norepinephrine, an immune suppressor. Dr. Larry Dossey, M.D. points out that thought and emotion affect the immune system at cellular and subcellular levels. [28]

Our immune system has a built-in intelligence, always correcting, altering course based on individual needs and conditions. It would be wise to start trusting the immune system, rather than assuming it is inferior until artificially "immunized."

> "We must begin by thinking health, rather than disease; of building or creating something desirable, rather than avoiding or destroying something undesirable. Freedom from illness is a by-product of thinking and building health, not of fighting diseases. It is more constructive to think of disease as something we build from within rather than something that attacks us from without." [29]

What If?

What if our culture chose to cling to the theories of Bechamp instead of Pasteur? Medicine would be "health" oriented rather than "disease" oriented. Instead of classifying microorganisms and disease entities, environments and life-styles would be classified. Instead of fighting germs, it would build health. In agriculture, it would not focus on killing pests but on building a balanced, healthy soil that can produce healthy plants that don't attract pests. [30]

Why do some people stay healthy while those around them get sick? How and why do we recover from disease after the cleansing action of fever? Why is the body revitalized following the detoxification of fasting? Why do some people suffer more from the same disease than others? Could there be one answer to all these questions (and more)? Could a mystery of life be revealed in how we think about health and disease? Did we make a mistake 130 years ago?

We have been taught to believe that germs are the body's ultimate enemy. This "germ theory" leads people to believe that they should not be responsible for their illness. It allows them to reject any notion other than being innocent victims of an arbitrary invasion, over which they had little control. The battle against disease breeds fear, and fear spreads when we think the war might be lost. Rejecting the traditional germ theory and embracing the ideas of Bechamp, reduces fear by giving back a sense of control and new hope for longer life and healthier living.

We could refer to our illnesses as imbalances we reap as a result of unwise choices, and not something that attacks us. "Instead of saying, 'I caught a cold,' why not say, 'I created a cold.'" [31]

THE BENEFITS OUTWEIGH THE RISKS?

On pure statistics, your child has a much greater chance of dying in a car accident (50,000 annually) than catching or dying from any of the childhood diseases combined. Simply taking the child in a car to the doctor is riskier than the chance of catching or dying from these childhood diseases. Suddenly, the perspective changes. So why are parents concerned about childhood diseases? What are the benefits of vaccination? What are the risks? We are led to believe that the benefits far outweigh the risks. But do they?

Statistics show how certain diseases decreased significantly *before* vaccines *or* antibiotics. However, vaccines are *assumed* to be responsible for the near lack of certain infectious diseases. If there is reasonable doubt whether vaccines can prevent epidemics, then the benefit side dims.

Since a person may or may not get a given disease in his or her lifetime, the *benefit* to that person *cannot* be measured. However, the *risks* to vaccination are undeniable: reaction, injury or death. They can be measured. They are tangible. Furthermore, there are *unknown* risks in vaccination. Vaccines have been implicated in a wide variety of chronic conditions.

If diseases, *even those for which no vaccine exists*, rise and fall on their own and if people who are vaccinated still get diseases vaccinated against, then society's benefit remains highly questionable. An unvaccinated person has *one* "risk" and that is of "catching" a disease. A vaccinated person has *two* risks: the chance

13

of "catching" the disease *plus* vaccine damage.

Since half of all disease cases (of measles and pertussis for example) occur in vaccinated people, then:

- for a vaccinated person who gets a disease, his benefit is 0% and his risk is unknown.

- for a vaccinated person who does not get a disease or a reaction, his benefit is unknown and his risk is unknown.

- for a vaccine-damaged or killed person, his benefit is 0% and his risk is 100%.

In subsequent chapters of this book, the reader will learn of specific vaccine failures and vaccine reactions for each of the childhood diseases. Reactions cannot be predicted prior to vaccinating — it's a chance that is taken every time. But society does not benefit by *one* child taking vaccine risk. We cannot be sure of the benefits of each vaccine, but *each* vaccine carries inherent risks, known and unknown. If the chances of certain diseases are so low then a parent choosing to protect his child from a perceived greater danger of possible vaccine-induced harm, cannot be faulted. Even though vaccines are deemed beneficial to society as a whole, parents make decisions about the welfare of their child based on the individual. In other words, "What will be the best for *my* child?" Working together, giving *each* child the best, eventually translates into a better society.

In the case of the pertussis vaccine where there are *at least* 1000 deaths per year from the vaccine and only 10 deaths from the naturally occurring disease, the *risks* far outweigh the benefits. [32]

Studies of the meningitis vaccine have shown it could be directly increasing rather than decreasing cases. Is any perceived benefit worth the risk of *inducing* disease or injury in a child? If diseases are the "enemy" is it not like *joining* the opposition by *making* someone sick?

It is truly impossible to give a clear benefit/risk analysis when the risks remain largely unknown. If they are unknown, risks *could* very well be huge, extremely disproportionate to any perceived "benefit," possibly making the risks of diseases by themselves appear rosy. With 95% of the population being vaccinated, the *potential* for negative effects could be *enormous*. So it could be *millions upon millions* of adverse effects vs. thousands of disease cases. So the *real* benefit/risk ratio, dependent upon *perceived* dangers, cannot be objectively determined.

WHY DO VACCINES APPEAR TO WORK?

- **Misleading Statistics**

- **Misinterpreting Antibody Count**

- **Misunderstanding of Vaccine Reactions**

- **True Immunity or Just Tolerance?**

Misleading Statistics

From 1850 to 1940, diseases had declined 90% and were at an all-time low, just when vaccines started to be introduced. [33] Antibiotics were not around until *after* this impressive decline, showing diseases's natural fall. In addition, diseases for which there was never a vaccine also declined dramatically. These huge reductions in disease prior to vaccines are due mainly to improvements in public and personal hygiene.

The reason most or all of the credit for "wiping out" infectious diseases goes to vaccines is that their introduction *coincided with a natural decline in disease.* Then, when a population is fully vaccinated, it becomes *impossible* to tell whether the disease declined because of the vaccines or would have anyway. There is evidence that might prove vaccines had little or nothing to do with a decline in disease. In countries without as widespread use of vaccines, and in diseases for which there is no vaccine, there was also a general decline.

The process of polio case reporting leaves questions as to how much this disease "declined" due to changes in reporting requirements (see polio chapter), not from the vaccine. In addition, the disease was already on a downward curve when the Salk vaccine was introduced. After repeated failure with this killed virus vaccine, the Sabin oral polio live virus vaccine was used instead, and by that time, the disease was showing a further decline anyway. Again, countries without such widespread use of the polio vaccine, also saw the disappearance of polio.

Statistics are used to show a decline in disease and because vaccines were introduced in the midst of this, credit, though misplaced, easily falls to the vaccines.

Misinterpreting Antibody Count

Certain people develop antibodies in their blood naturally. If this happens after having a disease or after being exposed to a disease, they are thought to be immune. There are those who don't develop antibodies and still never get certain diseases regardless of repeated exposure. They are also immune because their outer defenses are stronger.

With great hope of instilling immunity artificially, vaccines were developed because they *create* circulating antibodies in the blood. This is thought to be true immunity. But when the first-line-of-defense is bypassed, the blood stream is left to cope with foreign invasions (vaccines) all alone. It is questionable whether true immunity can be accomplished by totally skipping the body's designed initial response to antigens.

Antibody production in the blood remains the primary measure of vaccine efficacy. In other words, depending on the level of antibodies to a certain toxin in a vaccine, a person is determined to be immune to that disease. But prominent lab technicians say that the high antibody titre count has nothing to do with the prevention of any disease. Those with a high titre count often develop the worst cases of disease while those with the low count may or may not develop signs of illness. [34]

In *every* incidence of infectious disease, there are those exposed who never show signs or symptoms of that illness. Therefore, any person may or may not get a given disease in his lifetime, regardless of exposure to a disease, so you can't say he was "protected" from that disease only by the vaccine.

In 87 subjects with *naturally acquired immunity* to rubella, circulating immune complexes were *not* found. But in 39 out of 65 subjects vaccinated with attenuated rubella virus vaccine, circulating immune complexes *were* found. A large portion of *these* subjects suffered from arthralgias following vaccination in spite of their circulating "immune" complexes. [35]

When scientists were hoping to use antibody levels as a reliable standard for comparing different vaccines, they found they could not. Studies showed that the Japanese pertussis vaccine produced high levels of antibodies to that bacteria, which experts predicted would be correlated with the degree of protection from the disease. But a Swedish study found no such correlation. [36]

Another study investigated the relationship to the incidence of diphtheria to the presence of antibodies. The conclusion was that there was no relation whatsoever between the antibody count and the incidence of the disease. This study determined the existence or non-existence of antibodies in people who developed diphtheria and those who did not, but were in close proximity to those who did (such as physicians, nurses working in hospitals, family and friends). The researchers found people, who were highly resistant, with extremely *low* antibody counts and people developing the disease who had *high* antibody counts. [37]

The body's first-line-of-defense is the mucous membranes of the nose and mouth and the digestive tract. When these mechanisms are strongest, antigens (viruses, bacteria, foreign substances) never gain access to the blood stream, thereby never causing the development of antibodies. Antibodies are not produced when the primary immunological defenses are functioning at maximum capacity. In naturally occurring disease, the presence of antibodies could prove that the first-line-of-defense has *failed*. This would show a general weakness of that individual, allowing the disease to take advantage of his susceptibility. When a vaccine is given, the primary defenses are *automatically* averted. This may give assurances that a person is immune to a particular disease, when in fact his natural defenses were unable to meet the challenge properly, putting the rest of the immune system at a disadvantage.

The antibody response to a vaccine entering the blood occurs purely as an isolated technical feat, without any general inflammatory response (mechanism to rid the body of infection) or any noticeable improvement in overall health of the individual. [38] When doctors and others quote studies on how effective is this or that vaccine, very often the study is done purely on antibody production in the blood (eg: "This vaccine was shown to be 95% effective."). These statistics artificially inflate vaccine efficacy. Such methods clearly cannot be relied upon for proper scientific evaluation.

Misunderstanding Vaccine Reactions

Traditional vaccine theories consider severe reactions unfortunate but few, so they are justified. This provides false comfort to the vast majority who react mildly or not at all. The *absence* of a reaction to a vaccine could be due to one of two reasons. 1) If a child is extremely healthy (in our modern society this would be quite rare), the lack of a reaction may be because he is simply not sensitive due to the efficiency of his immune system, or 2) If the body is very weak, the defenses are *incapable* of producing an immediate reaction to the vaccine. [39] In this case, the body is left to adapt to the poisons and chances are it will remain susceptible to that disease, and in a weakened state, also susceptible to many others.*

More often, children experience mild reactions to vaccines.

---

*AIDS patients can often have full blown diseases and because their immune system cannot illicit the normal defenses, symptoms to a disease would not be apparent.

This is a sign that the body's defenses are responding to the influence of the vaccine. However, in the *mild* reaction, the defense is not strong enough to entirely deflect the effect of the vaccine. If the vaccine causes stronger symptoms such as fever, etc. the defense may be able to successfully counteract the influence of the vaccine. [40] This could explain why some show no measure of antibodies after a vaccine.

In the case of a very strong reaction with complications and possible permanent damage, the defenses are too weak to counteract the influence of the vaccine, so a deep illness is produced. If the person survives the complication, his state of health may remain impaired for a very long time. [41]

When severe reactions are few and mild reactions misinterpreted, vaccines are given undeserving credibility. Coupled with low incidence of diseases and few outward signs of vaccine reactions, people are led to believe that vaccines are doing the job for which they were intended. But no reaction means a child could still be susceptible to diseases, mild reactions prove the body is not properly ridding itself of infectious agents, and severe reactions are the result of an onslaught of poisons into a body that is totally unprepared to handle them. One could draw the conclusion that vaccines are only manipulating the immune system and not responding in ways calculated and predictable like vaccine scientists are leading the public to believe.

True Immunity or Just Tolerance?

Over half of all that is known about the immune system has been learned in the past 20 years or so. Rather than being simple, immune functions are now recognized as highly complex. The complexities could approach those of the brain and nervous system, the most intricate of all biological systems. [42]

How the immune system operates has been misinterpreted and misapplied. Accepted knowledge of one aspect of immunity conflicts with accepted knowledge of another aspect. For example, it is universally accepted that when a person is exposed to certain drugs over a long period of time (whether legal or illegal), higher and higher doses are required in order to achieve the same effect. Also, when a person is first exposed to alcohol, his tolerance is very low and the effects are felt much sooner. After a period of time, a person can "handle his liquor" and drink amounts that would put a tea-totaler unconscious. Nicotine displays a similar response. The first cigarette often makes a person sick; watery eyes, nausea, coughing are not uncommon. After a period of time, this person smokes one or two packs a day without many obvious *outward* effects. Are these "addicted" people *healthier* than those who do not use drugs, alcohol or cigarettes? Are these people considered *immune* to drugs, alcohol and cigarettes? Of course not. We say that these people can *tolerate* large amounts of poison, and if they don't cut down or quit, they can expect heart attacks, high blood pressure and cancer. These people no longer get sick from the *first* cigarette or drink but they are not healthier. They are more subject to the chronic, less curable and more devastating diseases.

The body does not build a defense to poison if given in small doses over a period of time. The body is never immune to poisons, just less and less capable of defending itself. The more the body is subjected to toxins, the less vital it becomes. [43] After repeated exposure to a poison, failure to resist is interpreted as immunity or neutralization, but this is not necessarily the case. [44] The body may be no longer able to respond to poisons with the usual acute symptoms because the toxin was driven deeper when the response became progressively weaker. [45]

True immunity is the body's ability to *resist* the influence of toxins, not merely *adapt*. With acute infections or exposure to toxins, the effort of resistance is vigorous, violent and exhausting. In chronic disease, *adaptations* have taken place in order to conserve vital energy. This adaptation is called tolerance. The body is capable of huge amounts of toleration, but at a cost. The body pays for this toleration by lowered resistance to every other influence. [46]

A person is said to be immune when, after exposure, he does not become ill with that disease. This is well-accepted medical thinking. *Immunity* is when the body *resists* infection. *Tolerance* is when the body adapts to repeated exposure to toxins. It is clear that vaccines are forcing the body to *adapt* (tolerate).

It is dangerously misleading to claim that a vaccine makes one "immune" or protects against an acute disease. Ironically, the same people who would agree that alcoholics and heavy smokers can *tolerate* high levels of toxins may interpret the body's apparent ability to "resist" infection from a disease because of vaccination, as true immunity. Just as a person is not "immune" to alcohol or cigarettes, his body may be actually *lacking* any ability to resist at all. The body's ability to defend itself and the body's overall health is greatest when toxins are tolerated least.

After the initial reaction to a vaccine, the virus that is left in the body is harbored *chronically*. All acute responses to the vaccine have ceased and the body is left to *adapt* to the remaining poisons. Through this adaptation, the body has been weakened to such a degree that these toxins are not effectively eliminated and *future* challenges to the immune system are not dealt with as efficiently. [47]

A tolerated high level of toxicity is the principal factor in producing chronic degenerative disease, and is always a factor in aging and curtailing life expectancy. The body cannot defend itself when vitality has been lowered to a point where it no longer has the energy and resources to conduct detoxification and healing processes. [48]

Vaccines may appear to "work" because after repeated "exposure" to the toxins of a vaccine, the body is less and less able to respond. But if the body is already undergoing an "attack" after vaccination, it cannot elicit the acute symptoms normally associated with that illness. This may *seem* like an accomplishment temporarily, but if years down the line, the body is finally able to rid itself of most of the poison, then it is once again susceptible to that very same disease. This is why we see some diseases such as measles postponed into the adolescent years. Were vaccinated victims of measles *ever* really immune to that disease, or were they just less able to muster an acute attack to rid the body of infection all at once?

What is wrong with a tolerance to acute diseases? It takes great amounts of energy to tolerate a poison, leaving the body weaker and more susceptible to chronic conditions. Vaccination assumes the body will be able to tolerate a few acute infections. The trouble with this theory is that the body is subjected to many more influences (toxins) than these few diseases, and it should be as vital as possible when encountering all of them. If scientific thought integrated knowledge about the immune system, vaccines would be seen as forcing the body to tolerate, exactly as in drugs, alcohol, smoking and other poisons, and *not* improving health or creating immunity.

WHAT IS IN A VACCINE?

To manufacture a vaccine, the disease must be grown in a culture and the bacteria or virus must be killed or inactivated, then the substance must be chemically preserved. The questions are: what is it grown in and what are the chemicals?

Manufacturers of vaccines admit they are highly toxic and by their very nature, cannot be made safe. [49] When cancer causing elements are found in foods, they are either banned (remember cyclamates?) or an obvious warning label appears on the package (saccharin, cigarettes). There seems to be a double standard for vaccines.

These are among the ingredients found in vaccines:

Phenol — (carbolic acid) a deadly poison.

Formaldehyde — a known cancer-causing agent which is commonly used to embalm corpses.

Thimerosal (a mercury derivative) — a toxic heavy metal that is not easily eliminated from the body.

Alum — a preservative.

Aluminum phosphate — used in deodorants. Toxic.

Aluminum and oil adjuvants — cancer-producing in laboratory mice.

Actone — a solvent used in fingernail polish remover. Very volatile.

Glycerin — a tri-atomic alcohol extracted from natural fats which are putrefied and decomposed. Some toxic effects of glycerine are kidney, liver, lung damage, diuresis, pronounced local tissue damage, gastrointestinal damage and death. [50,51,52]

Vaccines also will contain killed or diluted infectious organisms, solutions containing toxins of these organisms, or substances extracted from infectious agents. [53] Animal parts such as pig or horse blood, dog kidney tissue, monkey kidney tissue, chicken or duck egg protein, and other decomposing proteins are used to grow the viruses. [54, 55] In the early 1970's, a vaccine researcher Leonard Hayflick warned against the use of monkey tissue in the production of polio vaccines. The SV40 virus (similar to the AIDS virus and possibly indistinguishable), was found in the polio vaccine. The problem of virus contamination of monkeys was once so bad that 60% to 80% of monkeys used to make polio vaccine had to be rejected. The British now manufacture polio vaccine only with human cells, but most of the world's polio vaccine is still made from kidney tissue of African green monkeys and rhesus macaques. [56]

Besides the possible risk of transferring animal viruses to humans, which may or may not be hazardous, one must consider simply the danger of injecting animal proteins. Proteins by themselves cannot be used by the body. They must be broken down during the digestive process into amino acids before they can be taken into the bloodstream and become useful to the human body. If any protein enters the blood stream by any means other than the digestive tract, it becomes a strong poison. [57]

Many strict vegetarians may not realize that their children could be injected with animal protein. Also, those fighting against the cruelty of animals may have difficulty using vaccines when animals are routinely exploited in their manufacture.

Much worse than the possible cruelty to animals, Congressman Robert Dornan, R-California, has recently introduced a bill (HR622, the Parent Drug Awareness Act) into legislation that will require the labeling of all vaccines manufactured using fetal tissues! Unborn babies in the production of vaccines is appalling. (At press time more information is being gathered regarding which vaccines, etc.)

Product information listed in the *Physician's Desk Reference* (PDR) have warned against using a vaccine in a child sensitive (allergic) to thimerosal (mercury). How could one know if a child is "allergic" to a *known* poison before vaccinating? *The Journal of the American Medical Association (JAMA, 1990)* [58] refers to methods of testing children who have demonstrated egg allergies prior to the administration of MMR vaccine (the virus is cultured in egg). It states, "…it has become apparent that reactions to the MMR vaccine can occur in egg-allergic individuals." The American Academy of Pediatrics recommends that persons with a history of anaphylactic reactions (allergic) following egg ingestion should not be vaccinated until they have been skin tested. [59]

There is much concern in the medical literature of allergic reactions to a common *food* that is used in the manufacture of vaccines. What about *known carcinogens*? What about *obvious poisons*? We do not do skin tests to determine sensitivity to *poisons* prior to vaccinating.

The question of whether a vaccine works or not, of whether it is safe or not almost seems a worthless debate when examining exactly what goes into a vaccine.

WHAT DO VACCINES DO TO THE BODY?

- **Bypass the Natural Immune System**

- **Exhaust the Immune Capacity**

- **Alter the DNA and RNA**

- **Cause Chronic Diseases**

Bypass the Natural Immune System

When injected, the virus and all other vaccine components end up in the blood stream. This is an unnatural way of handling foreign material, contrary to all other forms of ingestion. As Dr. William Albrecht states: "If you take water into your system as drink, it goes into your bloodstream directly from the stomach. But if you take fats, they move into your lymphatic system. When you take other substances like carbohydrates and proteins, they go into the intestines, and from there are passed through to the liver, as the body's chemical censor, before they go into the blood and circulate throughout the body. Most vaccination serums are proteins [and contain other chemicals in addition] and are not censored by the liver. Consequently, vaccinations can be a terrific shock to the system." [60]

The liver is an organ designed to protect from foreign invasions of all types. When a vaccine enters the blood stream directly, it gives free access to the major immune organs and tissues without the benefit of the body's usual methods of getting rid of it. [61]

When bacteria, viruses and other foreign materials are breathed or swallowed, the first-line-of-defense is the mucous membranes. Invasions are partially neutralized before entering the stomach, for example. The digestion system further destroys invaders. If the antigen eventually enters the blood stream through this natural method, the white blood cells attack and neutralize foreign substances. When vaccinating, the first-line-of-defense is totally eliminated, putting the blood at a severe disadvantage in defending the body against potential hazards.

Exhaust the Immune Capacity

According to sophisticated research at the Arthur. Research Corporation, Tucson, Arizona and other centers, after vaccination, a substantial portion of immune bodies, (T-lymphocytes) becomes committed to the specific antigens in the vaccines. Having been committed, these lymphocytes become incapable of reacting or defending against other antigens, infections or diseases. [62, 63]

Every child is born with a finite ability to combat disease. This is his total immune capacity. Once a child experiences a particular disease, permanent immunity is extremely efficient, using probably 3% to 7% of the total immune capacity of an individual. In the case of routine childhood vaccination, it is likely that as much as 30% to 70% of the total immune capacity becomes committed. [64]

Researchers point directly to the relationship of vaccines to thymus gland damage and suggest that this might be part of the explanation for the present increase in degenerative diseases. Ongoing studies indicate that abnormalities in the production of thymosin are associated with a wide variety of immunodeficiency and autoimmune diseases. Patients with various types of cancer, leukemia, lupus erythematosis, and rheumatoid arthritis usually show impairment of their thymus-dependent immune system. [65]

These findings could indicate that a child's immunological reserves are substantially reduced due to standard vaccine programs. Far from producing a genuine immunity, a vaccine may actually interfere with or suppress the immune response as a whole, in much the same way that radiation, chemotherapy and cortocosteroids and other anti-inflammatory drugs do. [66]

Alter the DNA and RNA

Vaccines were introduced at a time of general ignorance of RNA and DNA molecular biology. Using viruses in vaccines, and animal tissue to culture them is a form of genetic engineering, over which has been considerable moral debate.

The genetic material of all living organisms, including viruses is either DNA or RNA. [67] American virologists have shown the RNA viruses, although not containing DNA material within their structure, are able to form DNA and become integrated with the cells that they infect. *Live attenuated viruses used for vaccines, implant foreign, alien material derived from animal culture tissues into the human genetic system.* [68]

Viruses are *immensely more powerful* than the characteristics of its given disease. They have the ability to change human genes and in the case of vaccination, actually incorporate animal genes into human cells. By their very nature, live viruses might be considered genetic messengers, made up entirely of DNA or RNA material. It would be difficult to conceive of more ideal agents than live viruses to serve as genetic carriers if we were attempting to bring about genetic transmutations in the human body. [69]

It is impossible to separate antibodies from the proteins of the animal in the making of vaccines. Further, there is no evidence that anti-toxins of one species can be made use of by another species. The injected germ proteins hybridize with the body proteins to form new tribes, half animal and half human, whose characteristics and effects cannot be predicted. [70]

Cause Chronic Diseases

With the present methods of the viral vaccines cultured in animal tissue, there is free exchange of genetic DNA and RNA, resulting in RNA-DNA hybridization. [71] Dr. Richard Moskowitz suggests that the vaccine may be incorporated into the body's own cells where it is capable of continually stimulating antibody production. Various kinds of naturally occurring viruses are stored within the cells of certain individuals and are associated with chronic diseases (herpes, tumors, panencephalitis). So it is conceivable that vaccines could cause similar occurrences if they are stored within the cells. Further, the constant sensitization of the immune system to the vaccine components within the body's own cells may weaken the natural ability to fight off *other* viruses and may cause serious problems. [72]

Although the body will not make antibodies against its own tissues, viruses becoming part of the genetic make-up may cause cells to appear foreign to the immune system making them a fair target for antibody production. [73] Because the antibodies cannot rid the body of the virus completely, the virus eventually succeeds in attaining a state of latency within the cell. The circulating antibody will thereafter keep the virus within the cell, preventing any acute inflammatory response. Antibodies could then begin to be produced in large quantities against the cells themselves. [74]

Under proper conditions these latent pro viruses could become activated and cause a variety of diseases including rheumatoid arthritis, multiple sclerosis, lupus erythematosis, Parkinson's disease and cancer. [75]

Artificial immunization has essentially traded off acute, epidemic diseases of the past century for the weaker far less curable epidemic of chronic diseases of the present. [76] If immune systems are being compromised by vaccines to such an extent that people cannot resist or overcome chronic diseases such as cancer and a myriad of other disabling and fatal conditions so rampant in our society, we may *wish* we had acute illnesses instead. Many of them are treatable and the death rates are lower than all chronic diseases. This "trade off" could *possibly* be justified except for the diseases we are supposed to be "protected from" still occur, in larger numbers than were probably expected.

.

Part II

Childhood Vaccines

PERTUSSIS (Whooping Cough)

Introduction

There is no childhood vaccine which is more dangerous or which causes more debate. The entire controversy usually revolves around the pertussis vaccine. It is very often the first to be decided against by parents and frequently starts the questioning of the safety and effectiveness of other vaccines, which forces this chapter into being the longest. There is much, much more about the dangers of the pertussis vaccine than could be included here. But as briefly as possible this chapter is meant to expose aspects of the disease and vaccine that are rarely found in the usual parent literature.

The Disease

Pertussis (commonly called whooping cough) is an infectious

and unpleasant disease but it is not the wide-spread killer it once was. During 1976-1985 there were four to eleven deaths associated with pertussis reported each year. [77] During 1986-1988 state health departments reported 10,468 pertussis cases. [78]

Pertussis had been falling steeply for 70 years prior to the vaccine. [79] Mortality rates continued to decline after the vaccine at a rate not significantly greater than before. [80]

There is a natural rise in pertussis cases every three or four years even in a vaccinated population and there is no evidence that the disease is milder in vaccinated children. [81]

The Pertussis Vaccine

The pertussis vaccine is usually given along with the diphtheria and tetanus vaccines (DPT). Every *week* about 67,000 children in the United States receive the DPT vaccine. [82] Children usually receive five doses before the age of seven.

The pertussis vaccine remains unchanged for nearly 50 years. [83] The American vaccine is called "whole-cell" because it is cultured or grown in large vats from whole cells of pertussis bacteria. The resulting vaccine contains endotoxins and pertussis toxin that remain active even after the bacteria that secretes them have been killed. Endotoxins are proteins secreted by a virus or bacteria that can affect the brain or produce shock. [84]

The amount of endotoxin in other consumer products are subject to strict federal regulation, but the regulations do not cover pertussis vaccine, in which endotoxins abound. There is 10,000 times as much endotoxin in pertussis vaccine than adults are allowed to receive in flu vaccines. [85]

Pertussis toxin is the other vaccine component responsible for neurological reactions. It can take longer to work on the nervous system causing reactions up to 30 days or more after a DPT shot. It is suspected of activating other allergic conditions. It might also suppress the immune system, making children vulnerable to infections. [86]

Pertussis toxin is highly toxic and scientists often use it to induce experimental brain damage in laboratory animals. To re-emphasize: when brain damage in laboratory animals needs to be induced, pertussis toxin is often used.

In 1985, 81 adults were accidently given the DPT. Seventy-five had reactions. Hard painful red lumps on their arms, fever, dizziness, chills, nausea, pain and suddenly elevated blood pressure were some effects of the vaccine. One was hospitalized for nine days. In proportion to body weight, a 10 pound infant receives *ten to twenty times* more pertussis vaccine than these adults. [87]

The whole-cell vaccine is not only crude and toxic, but also difficult to control. The potency of each vaccine lot varies even when produced by the same manufacturer. Labels carry standardized content information even though one vial of vaccine might be as much as 400% to 500% more toxic than another. [88]

The pertussis vaccine was developed in the mid 30's and was in wide-spread use by the late 1950's. [89] A pattern of infantile spasms that began appearing in medical literature in the 1940's is suspicious because it's the same decade that wide-spread pertussis vaccination was begun in the United States. [90] Since the 1940's there have been repeated reports by parents and medical researchers of children dying or being left with medication-resistant convulsions, mental retardation, learning disabilities and physical handicaps after reacting severely to a DPT shot. Yet despite four decades of evidence documented in the scientific literature of medical journals and books showing the history of reports confirming that the vaccine is highly reactive, there has not been any substantial improvements in the vaccine or the test used to screen the vaccine for safety. [91] In 1979, Sweden discontinued their pertussis vaccine because of public concern about severe adverse reactions and it was thought that the "protection" levels against pertussis were unacceptably low. [92] The medical literature is quick to point at Sweden's "soaring" rate of pertussis as a result of their not vaccinating. What is never mentioned is the death rate from the disease. Are the cases going up while the number of deaths remain the same? If so, then you could assume continued vaccination is this country is doing nothing to lower the number of deaths from pertussis. In the 1970's in England, Wales, and West Germany, vaccination was stopped and death rates actually fell. [93]

The Pertussis Vaccine Reactions

Some doctors will not give pertussis vaccine to their own children, others administer it in reduced doses in an effort to minimize possible adverse reactions. Most of the three and a half million children receiving the DPT shot every year in America will react mildly. What's worse is the department of Health and Human Services estimates that every year in the U.S., about a *half million* DPT shots are followed by reactions severe enough to contraindicate the administration of more pertussis vaccine. [94]

The only large study ever conducted in the United States found that one in 875 DPT *shots* is followed by a convulsion or shock/collapse episode. This means that 18,000 DPT shots annually may produce one of these two serious neurological reactions. Since most children will receive *five* shots, this could be converted to one in 3600 *children every year*. One Swedish study showed a rate of *permanent* brain damage or *death* in one in 17,000 children. [95]

Per year in the United States

(of children vaccinated with DPT):

- 35,000 *children* react with convulsions, collapse or high pitched screaming.

- 11,000 to 12,000 *children* react with seizures, shock or high pitched screaming which will probably go on to exhibit permanent neurological damage including developmental delay, learning disabilities, hyperactivity, behavior disorder, autism, epilepsy that cannot be controlled by medication and profound retardation. [96]

1981 British Study

(Most U.S. vaccine authorities rely on this study for statistics on the DPT)

- 1 in 110,000 DPT *shots* [1 in every 22,000 *children*] results in a serious neurological reaction.
- 1 in 310,000 DPT *shots* [1 in every 62,000 *children*] results in permanent brain damage. [97]

These figures are often misquoted by U.S. physicians as 1 in 110,000 *children*. Each child may receive three to five doses of vaccine, so these figures would be in error to a significant degree. Besides, to rely on this study is unscientific because the British uses a different whole-cell pertussis vaccine that appears to be less potent. Also, high risk children were excluded from this study even though these high risk children are routinely vaccinated in the United States. In addition to that, all reactions were not counted. The study counted only those children who were not hospitalized or who had a convulsion lasting 30 minutes or longer. Children can have convulsions lasting less than 30 minutes and still become brain damaged. The study's authors cautioned against using the reaction rate figures for other countries, but United States health authorities continue to use these figures even though it is probably a great underestimate of the actual risk for American children. [98]

Another Study

    37.7% had local redness
    40.7% had pain at the injection site
    50.9% had swelling at the injection site

UCLA/FDA Study

1 in 875 DPT *shots* resulted in a convulsion or collapse/shock reaction. Two babies in the study died following the DPT reaction symptoms but their deaths were classified as sudden infant death syndrome (SIDS). [99]

Rate of Reaction Per Number of Children

1 in 20: persistent crying
1 in 66: high fever
1 in 180: high pitched screaming
1 in 350: convulsions
1 in 350: shock or collapse
1 in 22,000: acute brain disorder
1 in 62,000: permanent brain damage
1 in 71,600: death [100, 101]

Vaccine critics say as many as 900 deaths and 12,000 cases of brain damage are due to the vaccine but are mistakenly attributed to other causes. One investigation said that *30% of SIDS babies* had exhibited classic vaccine reactions before they died a few days later. An estimate of *at least* 13% of all "unexplained" infant deaths occurring nationally can be attributed to the DPT vaccine. [102]

Each year between 6,000 and 15,000 babies die and their deaths are listed as SIDS. One study concluded that 17 of 23 vaccinated SIDS infants (or about 32%) died within one week of a DPT shot and six (or about 11%) died within 24 hours of the shot. A study in 1987 showed a 7.3 fold increase in cases of SIDS from zero to three days after immunization with the DPT vaccine. [102] Very often health officials will describe a death shortly after a DPT shot as "temporal" or coincidental. The trouble with this theory is that a population of babies and children with a vaccination rate of about 95% during their first year, there is no unvaccinated population with which to compare. The only proper comparison would be the death rate of a totally unvaccinated group of babies compared to a vaccinated group of babies. Comparing the population as a whole gives a "control group" of 95% vaccinated babies.

Most studies of adverse reactions limit their observation period. For example, it might be limited to two days following a vaccine. Some studies have extended this period to a week or two. [104] Delayed reactions do occur and are not included in most studies. So official damage and death estimates are probably much too low.

Official Categories of High Risk

[According to the vaccine manufacturers, The American Academy of Pediatrics (AAP) and The Advisory Committee on Immunization Practices (ACIP)]

The following puts a child at high risk of reacting to the pertussis vaccine and are considered reasons NOT to vaccinate:

1. Child is acutely sick with a fever or respiratory infection.

2. Child is taking medication that may suppress the immune system.

3. Child has a personal history of convulsions or neurological disease.

4. Child is past the seventh birthday.

5. Child had a severe reaction to a previous dose.

Suspected High Risk Categories

These categories are not officially recognized but they are listed in the vaccine literature as reasons NOT to vaccinate:

1. Child is ill with anything including a runny nose, cough, ear infection, diarrhea, or has recovered from an illness within one month prior to a scheduled DPT shot.

2. Child has a family member who has reacted severely to a DPT shot. There is strong evidence of genetic predisposition. Additionally, there have been reports of two, three and four pertussis vaccine damaged children in one family.

3. Child has a family history of convulsions or neurological disease. Many European countries including England, the Netherlands and Sweden advise against the pertussis vaccine if a member of the child's immediate family has a history of convulsions or seizure disorder.

4. Child was born prematurely or with low birth weight.

5. Child has had cerebral irritation in the neonatal period (such as trauma at birth from a difficult delivery; high

pitched screaming with arching of the back; or meningitis).

6. Child has a personal or family history of severe allergies (such as eczema, asthma and especially allergy to cow's milk).

Children with a history of convulsions are six times more likely to have an adverse reaction to the pertussis vaccine. But the 1975 World Health Organization stated that children from *families* with a history of neurological disorders should not be vaccinated either. This is not officially recognized by the AAP or the ACIP. They will say that children with a history of seizures or neurological disorders in the family *should* be vaccinated. The manufacturers hold otherwise. Lederle (American Manufacturer) says they shouldn't. Connaught (Canadian Manufacturer) says the question should be "carefully considered." [105] Every year, 198,000 American children will receive the pertussis vaccine despite their family histories of convulsions. [106] Listed in the medical literature as the *official* reasoning to continued vaccinations of high risk children is that if they were excluded, it would leave *too many children unvaccinated!*

The AAP and ACIP say it is safe to vaccinate a child with a minor illness. Manufacturers say it should be deferred. Lederle adds that parents should be asked about the child's recent health and questioned on the next visit about any signs of an adverse reaction to the previous dose. [107] This rarely occurs in practice.

Guidelines to identify children who should not be given DPT are often contradictory. Vaccine manufacturers generally give more conditions that put children at risk than either the American Academy of Pediatrics (AAP) or the Public Health Services' Advisory Committee on Immunization Practices (ACIP). Even the AAP guidelines are not consistently followed. Of 400 pediatricians and child neurologists who answered a questionnaire, 19% said they would reimmunize a child who cried persistently and inconsolably after a DPT shot, *even though the AAP's Red Book says they shouldn't.* [108]

Official Severe Reactions

The following severe reactions are recognized by the official vaccine policy-makers and are reasons NOT to give additional pertussis vaccine:

1. Allergic hypersensitive reaction. Hives, swelling of the mouth or throat, difficulty breathing, hypertension and shock within minutes or an hour of the shot.

2. Shock/collapse. About three hours after the shot the baby suddenly becomes marble white, cold and collapsed.

3. High pitched screaming or persistent crying for three hours or more.

4. High temperature. The product information inserts of one vaccine manufacturer considers a temperature of more than 103° to be a contradication to further pertussis vaccine.

5. Excessive sleepiness. A state of sleep which the infant cannot be aroused.

6. Convulsions.

7. Encepalopathy. Bulging fontanel, unusual unresponsiveness to parents, sudden eye crossing, inability to move an arm or leg, repetitive movements of any part of the body, negative change or regression in physical, emotional or intellectual behavior.

Suspected Severe Reactions

1. Severe local reaction. Pain, redness, soreness or swelling around the site of the injection. There have been reports of vaccine damaged children who had severe local reactions after a DPT shot and then followed by more involved systemic or neurological reactions after a subsequent shot.

2. General systemic reactions. These have been reported by parents of vaccine-damaged children: body rash, vomiting or diarrhea within hours of the shot, loss of appetite, loss of

weight, chronic diarrhea, ear and respiratory infections, new allergies.

3. Thrombocytopenia and hemolytic anemia. Two blood disorders which have been reported rarely following DPT shot.

4. Diabetes and hypoglycemia following vaccination. Infants who show serious reactions can suffer from failure to maintain glucose homeostasis. [Official Categories of High Risk, Suspected High Risk Categories, Official Severe Reactions, and Suspected Severe Reactions from *Whooping Cough, the DPT Vaccine and Reducing Vaccine Reactions* [109]].

Besides the debilitating or fatal reactions to DPT, a mother will often describe how her previously healthy child became chronically ill following a DPT shot. Suddenly the child is "never well" suffering from a constant runny nose, bronchial congestion and ear infections or the onset of allergies—all of which are resistant to antibiotics, antihistamines, and other medications. [110]

In defending the pertussis vaccine, many health authorities become trapped in a contradiction. On the one hand, they minimize and sometimes outright deny the significance of evidence linking the vaccine to serious events, including brain damage and death. But they keep limited statistics on these events, do risk-benefit calculations, support legislation to compensate vaccine victims and promote development of a safer vaccine. [111] These actions seem contradictory to their "official" position on the DPT vaccine.

Benefits/Risks

The benefits of the pertussis vaccine DO NOT outweigh the risks. There is a *94 times greater risk* of dying from the vaccine than from whooping cough itself. *There is a 3,888 times greater risk* of acquiring long term damage from the vaccine than from whooping cough itself.

The Vaccine Causes More Brain Damage Than Whooping Cough:

	Pertussis	Pertussis Vaccine
Death	10	943
Damage	3	11,666

There are about 10 deaths per year from the disease and at least 943 deaths per year from the vaccine. There are three cases of long term damage from disease per year but at least 11,666 cases of long-term damage per year from the vaccine. [112]

People who say that the benefits of the pertussis vaccine outweigh the risks of vaccine damage do not have all the facts.

There are only two manufacturers of the whole-cell vaccine: Lederle (American) and Connaught (Canadian). Over the last several years, other manufacturers dropped out of the market due to increased liability risks. Ten DPT lawsuits are settled every year for an average cost of $1 million.

Multi-million-dollar lawsuits against manufacturers of the DPT vaccine have created liability problems that have been followed by a series of massive price increases. In 1986 a single dose costs 25 times more than it did in 1982. The price went from forty-five cents to $11.40. By comparison, the vaccine against diphtheria and tetanus alone (DT) has remained at sixty-seven cents per dose since 1984. [113] In May of 1987 Lederle and Connaught dropped their price of DPT to $8.92. But Lederle says that the liability situation for the DPT vaccine remains extremely tenuous and unpredictable. [114] Lederle lost its insurance in July of 1986 and now has to cover its own liability costs. They seriously considered pulling out of the market after they could no longer get insurance. Connaught has had its commercial insurance drastically curtailed and describes itself as "effectively self-insured." [115]

The Pertussis Vaccine Failures

"Epidemics" of pertussis have been reported after public

rejection of the vaccine but when scrutinized more closely, as in an analysis of a 1983 Maryland study, cases were in one of three categories almost exclusively: 1) bacteriologically unproven cases, 2) children under 2 months of age and not even eligible for DPT and 3) cases in children who were completely vaccinated. [116]

Most whooping cough in America today occurs in vaccinated children or those too young to be vaccinated. Only 37% of cases overall occur in unvaccinated children. [117] The state of Washington reported 162 cases in ten months in 1984 and 49% of the cases aged 3 months to 6 years had been appropriately vaccinated for their age with DPT. [118]

Today between 1,000 and 4,000 cases of whooping cough are reported to the Centers for Disease Control (CDC) annually. However, there may actually be 20,000 to 60,000 cases each year because the CDC estimates that the disease is under-reported in America by as much as 20 times. When an increase in pertussis is noted, it is possible that these are not real increases but simply a result of increased reporting of the portion of the 20,000 to 60,000 pertussis cases that are estimated to occur every year but have historically remained unreported. [119]

The overall problem of reporting can lead to the belief that the pertussis vaccine is more "effective" in preventing the disease than is actually the case. *The Morbidity and Mortality Weekly Report (1990)* reported that "diagnostic limitations restrict assessment of the full public health impact of pertussis." [120] The article suggests that the standard culture test (DFA) for diagnosing pertussis has a positive predictive value of 56% and should not be relied on for diagnosing and reporting pertussis. A child could have pertussis while a test comes back negative, resulting in the case going unreported.

Approved clinical diagnosis is a cough illness lasting more than 14 days, paroxysms, whoop, or post-tussive vomiting. The article goes on to say only "51% (in a 1984 survey of state and territorial epidemiologists) counted physician-reported pertussis if laboratory studies were not done. With such reporting practices, half the patients meeting the clinical case definitions may go unreported if laboratory tests are negative or not done." [121] This could lead to an overall impression that there are fewer cases of pertussis. Under-reporting of pertussis can reflect that the vaccine "works" more often than it "does" because there are fewer cases perceived.

It is known that at least half of all pertussis cases occur in partially or fully vaccinated individuals. Very often when a doctor knows a child has been vaccinated against pertussis, he will not culture for whooping cough and therefore that case of "vaccine failure" will go unreported. If all the unvaccinated cases were reported and few of the vaccinated cases were reported, it would lead to believing that the vaccine "works." In reality, there could be an even greater disproportion of vaccinated children getting pertussis.

Often adults and teenagers can have atypical whooping cough and only exhibit symptoms similar to a bad cold or flu. [122] These undiagnosed adult and teenage carriers of whooping cough, most of whom have been fully vaccinated, are not counted as vaccine failures.

Pertussis vaccine failures are hidden by the following factors:

1. An inaccurate test for pertussis leads to under-reporting of cases.

2. CDC estimates pertussis is actually 20 times higher than reported.

3. Only half of physicians may report clinical cases of pertussis. In addition, doctors may not culture in a suspected case of pertussis when the child was previously vaccinated.

4. Under-reporting suppresses pertussis cases, leading to belief in a vaccine that "works" less often than is perceived.

If all actual cases of pertussis were reported, the vaccine failures would become increasingly more obvious and faith in the vaccine would wane.

Also, physicians may diagnose whooping cough in an unvaccinated child when the disease is actually allergic bronchitis, influenza or atypical viral pneumonia. A number of other bacteria such as B. parapertussis, B. bronchoseptica, chlamydia, mycoplasma pneumonia, and various adenoviruses cause symptoms similar to pertussis. [123]

Reporting of vaccine *reactions* has similar problems. It is difficult to get exact figures for the United States because we look to doctors to provide accurate data on the incidence of disease as much as the incidence of adverse reactions to vaccines. [124] Most doctors either ignore, or are unaware of any requirement to report adverse reactions. Even when anxiety persuades parents to call their doctors about reactions, they are sometimes treated as "hysterical mothers" and reassured that "everything will be fine." [125]

Some doctors insist that reactions are coincidental and not due to the DPT shot at all. In that case, they obviously won't be inclined to report any reactions. With many parents and doctors opting for the DT (without pertussis) in certain children, simply by the large number receiving the DT vaccine only, suggests far more reactions to the DPT than are reported to the state health departments by doctors. [126]

To Sum It Up

☐ The incidence of pertussis had been falling steeply for 70 years prior to the vaccine.

☐ At least half of all pertussis cases are in vaccinated individuals.

☐ Severe under-reporting of this disease leads to false confidence in the vaccine.

☐ The pertussis vaccine reactions are the most severe of all the childhood vaccines.

☐ There is no solid agreement in policy or practice between manufacturers, vaccine policy-makers, and doctors on each: high risk categories, vaccine reactions, and contraindications to further doses.

☐ Multi-million dollar law suits against vaccine manufacturers for damage and death have raised the cost of vaccines substantially, caused other manufacturers to leave the market and caused the government to enact the Vaccine Compensation Act.

☐ The "benefits" of the vaccine DO NOT outweigh the risks!

ACELLULAR PERTUSSIS VACCINE

The Vaccine

Though not available in the United States, Japan has introduced a new and "safer" vaccine. The Japanese vaccine is "acelluar" in which the bacteria are removed, leaving bacteria fragments (whole-cell vaccines contain the dead bacteria cells and active toxins). In acellular, 95% of the endotoxins are removed leaving chemically deactivated pertussis toxin. [127]

A small number of pediatricians in California are risking their medical licenses to vaccinate children with this "safer" Japanese pertussis vaccine not FDA approved. The United States is far behind other countries in efforts to make a "safer" vaccine.

The Acellular Vaccine Reactions

In Japan, the new acellular vaccine resulted in a 60% reduction of "mild" side effects. But the rate of severe reactions did not differ significantly between the acellular and the traditional whole-cell vaccine. [128]

The Japanese are vaccinating children 24 months or older and scientists question whether the lower reaction rate is due to later vaccination or the vaccine itself. [129] However, a Swedish study did report severe systemic reactions with the acellular vaccine in infants. Of 212 infants receiving the acellular vaccine, two had serious reactions. These reactions are identical to those following the whole-cell vaccine. [130] This shows a serious reaction rate of 1 in 100, much higher than the reported rate in infants receiving the whole-cell vaccine.

The Acellular Vaccine Failures

Scientists question whether there is enough naturally occurring pertussis to accurately determine in clinical trials whether a new vaccine is effective or not.

As with any other vaccine, the full ramifications cannot be known for many years. The "safety" and "effectiveness" cannot be determined in the laboratory. Thousands of children receive vaccines on an "experimental" basis because the results are impossible to determine prior to widespread use.

To Sum It Up

☐ The new acellular pertussis vaccine does not seem to reduce severe reactions.

☐ It is questionable whether the vaccine's "safety" and "effectiveness" can be determined in the near future.

DIPHTHERIA

The Disease

There were between 0 and 5 cases of diphtheria per year reported in the United States during the 1980's. [131] Diphtheria can be found in throat cultures from individuals never showing symptoms of the disease. So, diphtheria is around but not causing widespread disease.

The Diphtheria Vaccine

The diphtheria vaccine is usually administered along with the pertussis and tetanus (DPT) or along with the tetanus vaccine only (DT). A child usually receives 5 doses before the age of seven.

The Diphtheria Vaccine Reactions

According to the *1990 Physician's Desk Reference*, the possible reactions to this vaccine (DT) include: subcutaneous atrophy at the site of the injection, drowsiness, fretfulness, vomiting, anorexia, persistent crying, pallor, coldness, hyporesponsiveness, convulsions, encephalopathy, Guillain-Barre syndrome, urticaria, erythema, arthralgias and anaphylactic reactions.

In Poland, researchers reported that 13 of 17 children who were given DT showed significant changes in their electroencephalograms. Seizure activity occurred for the first time or intensified previously present seizure activity. [132]

The Diphtheria Vaccine Failures

Diphtheria has occurred in vaccinated individuals. One recent report from the United States found that 1 of 3 diphtheria fatalities and 14 of 23 carriers of the organism were among fully vaccinated individuals. [133]

During about 1965 to 1980, the same death rate and the same severity of illness was found among the vaccinated and unvaccinated. [134]

Vaccination appears to have increased diphtheria in many countries. At the beginning of World War II, Germany made diphtheria vaccination compulsory. The diphtheria rate soared to 150,000 cases in 1939. At the same time in unvaccinated Norway, there were only 50 cases. In Paris, diphtheria rose as much as 30%. In Hungary, vaccination had been compulsory since 1938 and the diphtheria rate rose 35% in two years. In the Canton of Geneva vaccination had been enforced since 1933 and the number of cases tripled from 1941 to 1943. [135] Most French children had been vaccinated by 1941 and there were 13,795 cases by the end of that year. Shots were continued and by 1943 diphtheria cases were more than tripled to 46,750 cases. Official military records of the United States show that thoroughly vaccinated soldiers have a four times higher disease and death rate from the disease than do the unvaccinated civilians. [136]

After abandoning the diphtheria vaccination in Germany, the rate of diphtheria fell dramatically from 1946 to 1951. This was in spite of post-war overcrowding, poverty, undernourishment and general societal upheaval. In Sweden, without any diphtheria vaccination there was a virtual disappearance of the disease. The decline of diphtheria in Canada, a highly vaccinated country, was no faster than the rapid decline in Japan after 1945, and Japan never vaccinated for diphtheria. [137]

To Sum It Up

☐ Cases of diphtheria in this country are virtually non-existent.

☐ Reactions to the vaccine can be severe.

☐ Diphtheria has occurred in vaccinated individuals.

☐ The decline of diphtheria worldwide happened no faster in countries with vaccines than in countries without diphtheria vaccines.

☐ Diphtheria vaccination appears to have historically increased cases of diphtheria.

TETANUS (Lockjaw)

The Disease

Of the diseases children are normally vaccinated against, this disease is probably the most responsible for fear in parents. Many otherwise "non-vaccinators" give their child this vaccine only. Even though there are very few cases of tetanus, we are made to believe that our injury-prone young ones are at great risk. We might assume that once a person gets tetanus he has a 50-50 chance of surviving. Facts are, the death rate for those under 20 years old is 5%. [138] This chapter will attempt to dismiss the myths of this disease.

Though there are many more cases of tetanus world-wide, it may relieve parents to know that these are usually due to a lack of cleanliness. Thirty percent of world cases are associated with contaminated umbilical stump infections. [139]

Tetanus is a disease of the central nervous system produced by infection with the anaerobic bacteria (thrives in the absence of air) found in soil, dust, water, and intestinal tracts and fecal matter of humans and animals. So, a "rusty nail" *alone* cannot cause tetanus. Also, tetanus infects only wounds that contain dead tissue. [140] It is not contagious. It incubates from three days to three weeks or longer. [141] Since 1977, the incidence has continued to decline. [142]

There were 48 cases of tetanus reported in the United States in 1987 and 53 cases in 1988. Of these 101, ninety-nine had case details. Incidence increased with age. Sixty-seven of the 99 patients were more than 50 years old. Six were less than 20 years old. The youngest patient to contract tetanus in 1987 to 1988 was 2 years old. Fourteen of 99 cases were associated with chronic wounds or underlying medical conditions such as skin ulcers, abscesses or gangrene. Ten of these occurred in patients with diabetes. [143]

From 1985 to1986, seven cases, representing 5% of all tetanus cases in the U.S. were less than 20 years old. [144] And of those cases, the fatality rate was 5%. The majority of tetanus cases are people over 50 and their case-fatality rate is about 30%. [145]

So, statistically speaking, older adults are at greater risk of contracting tetanus than children and when contracted by a child, the death rate is much, much lower.

It is interesting to note the low incidence of tetanus as compared to a few other notifiable diseases:

US cases, 1989

Toxic-shock syndrome 362

Typhoid fever 465

Malaria 1,203

Tuberculosis .... 20,563 (1,800 deaths) [146]

Tetanus .... 53 (about 10 deaths, 1988) [147]

Your child has a much greater chance of catching and dying from the highly contagious disease of tuberculosis, than getting tetanus. Considering that there are about 50,000 fatal motor vehicle accidents per year, a child is more at risk in a car than at risk of dying from tetanus.

Good wound care is probably the single most important factor in the prevention of tetanus. Proper cleansing and removal of all foreign bodies and dead tissue can convert fresh tetanus-prone wounds to non-prone wounds. [148]

The Tetanus Vaccine

The tetanus vaccine is usually administered along with the

pertussis and diphtheria vaccines (DPT). It is also given with just the diphtheria vaccine (DT). A child usually receives 5 doses before the age of seven.

The Tetanus Vaccine Reactions

The possible side effects from this vaccine include: subcutaneous atrophy at the site of the injection, fever, rash, drowsiness, fretfulness, vomiting, anorexia, persistent crying, pallor, coldness, hyporesponsiveness, brachial plexus neuropathy (which can lead to paralysis of the arm), anaphylaxis (a form of shock), convulsions, encephalopathy, Guillain-Barre syndrome, urticaria, erythema, arthralgias and anaphylactic reactions. [149, 150]

In Poland, researchers reported that 13 of 17 children who were given DT showed significant changes in their electron-encephalograms. Seizure activity occurred for the first time or intensified previously present seizure activity. [151]

The Tetanus Vaccine Failures

In the two years between 1987 and 1988, six tetanus cases occurred in those less than 20 years old. Of these six, one had received one dose and three had completed the primary series of vaccines (3 doses), before they got the disease. So, the vaccine failed to "protect" in four out of six cases. Of the 85 patients total who received tetanus immune globulin after disease onset, 15 died. [152]

Since at least 40% of adults in this country don't get their "required" booster shots said necessary in order to "protect" them from tetanus, then it seems like we should be seeing many more cases of tetanus. [153] So, if a relatively unvaccinated adult population is still safe from tetanus, could we not assume an unvaccinated child population would be as safe?

To Sum It Up

☐ Parents should keep the disease, tetanus in perspective when contemplating the vaccination decision. Ask whether fear of this disease is merely because of the existence of a vaccine.

☐ Adults have a greater chance of contracting and dying from tetanus, but the focus remains misplaced on children.

☐ Some people who get tetanus have been previously vaccinated and some previously vaccinated people die from tetanus.

☐ Good wound hygiene is the best protection from the anaerobic bacteria of tetanus.

RUBELLA (German Measles)

The Disease

During 1988, 221 cases of rubella were reported. Rubella is a milder form of measles. It usually lasts only three days and natural infection results in life-long, permanent immunity to another occurrence. This disease is very rarely complicated and prior to vaccines, was considered among the harmless childhood illnesses.

Vaccination of all children is rationalized by the hope of preventing a woman from contracting rubella during the first three months of pregnancy, to reduce the chance of causing congenital rubella syndrome, or birth defects. In 1987, three cases of congenital rubella syndrome were reported and one in 1988. [154]

The Rubella Vaccine

The rubella vaccine was licensed in the United States in 1969. [155] The vaccine is derived from a human diploid (WI-38) cell culture. [156] It is usually given to children at 15 months of age along with the measles and mumps vaccines (MMR). It is also given to women of childbearing age who show no immune factors to rubella in blood tests. The recommended ages and doses are changing due to repeated vaccine failures (see Measles chapter).

In other countries, German measles vaccine is given in puberty, allowing for the natural possibility of the child to acquire life-long immunity. This vaccine remains controversial throughout the Western world. Little agreement has been reached on what age group should be vaccinated.

The Rubella Vaccine Reactions

The researcher who helped develop the first German measles vaccine refused to use it on his own children because he felt another vaccine had fewer side effects.

As reported by the *Journal of the American Medical Association (Feb. 20, 1981)*, OB-GYN physicians held the lowest vaccination rate. Of those known by blood test to be "susceptible" less than 10% submitted to vaccination. The next lowest rate of cooperation occurred among pediatricians. "Fear of unforeseen vaccine reaction" was the conclusion. Particular concern was over the Guillian-Barre syndrome seen with the influenza vaccine. [157] The people showing the lowest rate of vaccine participation are those expected to care the most about women's and children's health.

According to an article in *Science* in early 1970 the HEW reported that "as much as 26% of children receiving rubella vaccine in national testing programs developed arthralgia and arthritis." Many had to seek medical attention and some were hospitalized to test for rheumatic fever and rheumatoid arthritis. [158]

Other possible reactions include: encephalitis-type symptoms, meningitis, and Guillain-Barre syndrome (muscle paralysis and sensory nerve deficits); joint pain occurs in about 40% of those vaccinated; aches and pains or slight rash (a lot like the disease itself). [159]

Women who are vaccinated after puberty often experience swollen lymph glands, aches and pains and temporary arthritis. [160] These problems are more prominent and last longer than in younger children. [161] At least 12% to 20% of women develop arthritis symptoms after receiving the vaccine. These may begin several weeks after the administration of the vaccine. [162] They may persist for weeks, months or years. In some cases, women develop rheumatoid arthritis which continues throughout their lives. [163]

Another report says that in *20% to 40%* of adults receiving the live rubella vaccine, arthralgia and arthritis have been observed. Thrombocytopenia has been observed following the use of rubella vaccine, sometimes severe enough to be associated with purpura. [164]

The Rubella Vaccine Failures

It was published in the Congressional record in October of 1971 that the vaccine was released along with vaccines for measles, mumps and influenza for massive public programs without sufficient testing. [165]

With so many children being vaccinated, you would expect to see an ever-increasing immune adult population. But the rubella vaccine does not impart permanent immunity. Prior to the time of vaccination against rubella, 85% of adults were naturally immune to the disease. Now we see a much lower percentage. This suggests that vaccines are actually interfering with the population's ability to resist this infection. There are also reports of rubella in individuals who were appropriately vaccinated.

The *Medical Journal of Australia* reported a case where a rubella injection failed to prevent congenital rubella. In the U.S. during 1970 to 1980 (after wide-spread vaccination with rubella vaccine), one type of birth defect associated with rubella was *increased* by 300%. [166]

Rubella vaccination may be increasing the chance of infection in childbearing years because a large portion of children are found to have no evidence of immunity in blood tests four or five years after rubella vaccination. The reinfection rate can be as high as 80% compared with 4% in naturally immune individuals. [166]

During the three-year period before vaccine licensure (1966-1968), 23% of rubella cases occurred among people more than 15 years of age. In 1987, 48% of cases occurred in persons more than

15. [168] Are we seeing a reversal that forces cases into childbearing age, where the danger from the disease is greater to the adult and the unborn baby? The proposed solution to avert this problem of shifting age occurrence has been to revaccinate "susceptible" women of childbearing age. The question is, if the vaccine "wears off" then are we constantly shifting to an older and older population? Does this suggest that vaccinating all children is unnecessary?

To Sum It Up

☐ Rubella is a very mild disease in children.

☐ The rate of congenital rubella syndrome is almost zero.

☐ Neurologic reactions and arthritis have been reported following rubella vaccination.

☐ Childhood vaccination against rubella has shifted the occurrence of the disease into adolescence and women of childbearing age.

☐ The disease occurs in vaccinated individuals and congenital rubella has occurred in spite of vaccination.

MUMPS

The Disease

In 1987, there were over 12,000 reported cases of mumps. Mumps in children is not harmful. [169] Thirty to 40% of natural mumps are symptomless. [170] A natural case of mumps confers permanent immunity even in those cases which go unnoticed. Infection of the testicles, ovaries and other organs are not unusual but occur more commonly in adults. Sterility following mumps is *extremely* rare, and usually affects only one testicle. Mumps can be more serious in adults and it is thought that the mumps vaccine can create a tolerance that only postpones a more severe attack in puberty or adulthood. [171]

The Mumps Vaccine

A live mumps vaccine was licensed in 1967 and recommended for routine use in 1977. [172] It is usually given along with the measles and rubella vaccine (MMR) at the age of 15 months. However, due to the increase in measles cases over the last few years, recommended ages and doses are changing (see Measles chapter).

The Mumps Vaccine Reactions

The mumps vaccine is associated with side effects similar to the measles vaccine and includes: fevers, seizures, encephalitis and severe, atypical mumps disease. [173] The Centers for Disease Control reports the following side effects from the mumps vaccine: inflammation of the parotid glands, effects on the central nervous system such as febrile seizures, unilateral nerve deafness, and encephalitis within 30 days of mumps vaccination. [174] The most common reaction is meningitis caused by the mumps component of the MMR vaccine. [175]

The Mumps Vaccine Failures

One pediatrician was reported to have told the mother of a child who contracted mumps (in spite of his being previously vaccinated) that in his practice, he sees at least one case in every seven in previously vaccinated children. In other words, the vaccine fails to "protect" from mumps.

At least one report confirms that it is the vaccine strain itself and not the wild virus that causes vaccine-related mumps meningitis. Virus from the cerebrospinal fluid 21 days after immunization was identical to the vaccine strain. Nine cases pointed out that the incubation period of natural mumps infection was like that of vaccine-associated meningitis, often about 21 days. [176] If the vaccine can *induce* mumps meningitis then its value as a mumps "preventative" is questionable.

To Sum It Up

☐ Mumps is not a harmful disease in children.

☐ The mumps vaccine can cause more severe atypical cases of mumps and is associated with an increase in adolescent and adult cases, where the disease is more serious.

☐ There are adverse side effects associated with mumps vaccine including vaccine-associated meningitis.

☐ Previously vaccinated children can still get mumps, but a natural case confers permanent immunity.

MEASLES (Rubeola)

The Disease

Prior to the introduction of vaccines, measles, mumps, and rubella were among the routine childhood diseases which most school children contracted before the age of puberty and from which nearly all recovered uncomplicated, with permanent life-long immunity. Measles can be a devastating disease when a population encounters it for the first time. However, measles has become common in our population and it hardly deserves mention with other diseases associated with some vaccines. [177]

Complications such as pneumonia following measles must be kept in perspective. Measles does not *cause* pneumonia, rather it can be a complication, as it can be after *many other diseases.*

From 1958 to 1966 (before the live vaccine) the number of measles cases reported each year dropped from 800,000 to 200,000. [178] Recently, incidences have declined from an average of 40,000 reported cases per year in the 1970's to an average of 3,000 per year in the 1980's. [179] After reaching an historical low of 1,497 cases in 1983, the number of reported measles cases reached 6,282 cases in 1986 and more than 14,000 cases in 1989.

The Measles Vaccine

The killed measles vaccine was introduced in 1963. Atypical measles developed as a result of this vaccine. [180] In 1968, it was replaced with a live attenuated vaccine.

Measles, mumps and rubella vaccines (MMR) are usually given at 15 months of age. In 1969, the age for vaccine administration became 12 months, after vaccine failures in younger children. Because of continued vaccine failure, the age was raised again to 15 months. When statistics during a 1988 epidemic in Los Angeles showed that 38% of the cases were less than 16 months old, the age for vaccine administration was lowered again to 9 months in areas where measles was recurrent. These children would then require revaccination at 15 months of age. [181] Now, due to measles outbreaks in highly vaccinated populations, a second dose is recommended for school-age children.

The Measles Vaccine Reactions

Thrombocytopenia has been observed following the rubeola (measles) vaccine, sometimes severe enough to be associated with purpura. The number of cases of subacute sclerosing panencephalitis (SSPE) associated with *natural* rubeola virus has been *decreasing* and an *upward trend* has been observed in association with rubeola *vaccine*. [182] Other possible reactions include: encephalopathy, fever with rashes for five days in 15% of those vaccinated, retardation, ataxia, aseptic meningitis, seizure disorder, [183] malaise, sore throat, headache, nausea, erythema, regional lymphodenopathy, optic neuritis, retinits, ocular palsie, Guillain-Barre syndrome [184] and the current epidemic of hyperactivity in children have been associated with the measles vaccine. The vaccine can also destroy the protective sheath covering the nerves, brain and spinal cord. [185]

Atypical measles has occurred in children previously vaccinated. This consists of an illness with exaggerated rash, muscle weakness, peripheral edema and severe abdominal pain with persistent vomiting. [186] These reactions have also occurred following the vaccine. [187]

Research at Rutgers University shows live virus vaccines used against common ailments like influenza or measles may set the stage for a variety of diseases later. A certain enzyme portion of viruses may invade the genetic make-up of a vaccinated person. It may reappear later as multiple sclerosis, arthritis or even cancer. Over a long period, complications from the vaccine may occur and take a disease course that is not suspected when the vaccine was given. [188]

The Measles Vaccine Failures

A national goal was set to eliminate measles by 1982. Repeated reports of measles in fully vaccinated individuals and in highly vaccinated populations has foiled that plan.

- A review of measles outbreaks in the U.S. during 1985 to1986 revealed that a median of 60% of cases in school-age children occurred in *vaccinated* individuals. [189]

- Between January 1 and September 2, 1986, a sustained outbreak of 235 cases of measles-like rash illness occurred in Dane County, Wisconsin. Over 96% of enrolled students had school records of prior measles vaccination. [190]

- Of the 3,411 reported cases in the U.S. in 1988, 1,942 occurred among school-aged children. Of these, 68.9% had been appropriately vaccinated. [191]

- A review of 1,600 cases of measles in Quebec, Canada, between January and May, 1989 showed that 58% of school-age cases had been previously vaccinated. [192]

- In an outbreak of measles in Hobbs, New Mexico, 98% of the cases had been previously vaccinated. [191]

- In states with comprehensive vaccination requirements,

between 61% and 90% of measles cases occur in people who were appropriately vaccinated. [193]

These failure statistics may even be on the low end of the scale. According to an article in *JAMA, May, 1990*, "In an era when physicians are relatively unfamiliar with the disease, failure to detect measles in some vaccinated people will lead to 'calculation of artificially low attack rates' for the vaccinated population." [194] This will result in coaxing officials to believe that the measles vaccine is more "effective" than it is.

In at least one study, there were primarily two types of outbreaks of measles: those among highly vaccinated (vaccine coverage more that 90%) school-aged children and those among unvaccinated pre-school aged children. Now, a two-dose measles vaccine is recommended — the first at 15 months and the second dose later, in order to overcome the primary vaccine failure. The American Academy of Pediatrics recommends this second dose at age 11 or 12. The Centers for Disease Control (CDC) recommends this dose at entry to kindergarten or first grade (4 to 6 years old). Neither of these policies have been evaluated in any studies. [196]

The issue of second-dose measles vaccine warrants some scrutiny. Health officials are saying the first dose didn't work, so they are recommending a second dose at a later age. Yet, there are no studies that would give anyone even the slightest confidence that this would "work" either. If the first dose didn't work, why would the second? Also, if we are seeing measles in highly vaccinated adolescents and unvaccinated preschoolers, with virtually little difference in the rates, then could it be said that the first dose at 15 months was completely unnecessary? And is the second dose likely to be any more effective than the first dose when the medical literature refers to "waning vaccine immunity" as the cause of measles in vaccinated populations?

To put it more succinctly: when the question was asked during a three day meeting in Atlanta at the Centers for Disease Control, as to what data was available to support the belief that no serious adverse reactions will occur from revaccination, the answer was, "There is no data." [197]

To Sum It Up

☐ Measles is usually mild in children.

☐ There are many adverse reactions associated with the measles vaccine.

☐ At least 60% (often more) of the measles cases occur in previously vaccinated individuals.

☐ Due to recent outbreaks of measles in highly vaccinated populations, medical literature admits to the possibility of vaccine failure in a large portion of vaccine recipients.

☐ There is no consistent policy for the second-dose measles vaccine and there is still no proof of the safety or effectiveness.

POLIO

The Disease

There are three kinds of polio, ranging from a mild feverish illness lasting 24 to 48 hours to a severely crippling disease. [198] In 90% to 98% of illness associated with polio virus, it is inapparent or similar to common colds or flu characterized by sore throat, headache, nausea and abdominal pain. [199, 200] Only one kind causes paralysis. Paralytic polio begins in the same way and after a few days of minor illness, it is followed by a few days of well-being, then the same and more severe symptoms. After a period of days and weeks, return of muscle power begins and usually reaches its limits in 18 months. [201] Two to 10% of the *paralytic* cases are fatal and the death rate increases with age. [202]

Natural immunity to polio virus was already as close to being universal as it could be and no artificial substitute could approximate that result. Before the vaccine was introduced, the polio virus could be found routinely in samples of city sewage. [203] For every clinical case of polio, over 100 people got it without ever knowing it. [204] In underdeveloped countries where sanitation is poor, almost 100% of these children develop antibodies due to infection in infancy. Epidemics are unknown, paralytic cases are few, and the great majority are minor illnesses. [205]

Since polio causes a remarkably small number of cases resulting in death or permanent disability, a peculiar anatomical susceptibility may exist. [206] Also, some suggest that susceptibility to polio was increased by lowering natural resistance after the introduction of refined foods, environmental chemicals, modern drugs and vaccinations (of all kinds) on a nation-wide scale. [207] Perhaps the polio epidemics in the 1940's and 1950's marked the decrease in breast-feeding as mothers chose the bottle. Since mother's milk contains a neutralizing agent that inactivates the polio virus in the intestines of a child while breast feeding, [208] this could explain a rise in polio during that same period. As quoted in the *Physician's Desk Reference (PDR) 1990*, "it may be prudent to recommend abstention from breast-feeding for two to three hours before and after oral vaccination to permit the establishment of the vaccine viruses in the gut."

Since dental caries parallel polio, sugar can be implicated in causing or contributing to polio epidemics. During the years of epidemics, a rise in polio cases was always noted in the summer months, thus the public beach closures, etc. It is interesting to note that these months coincide with a huge increase in the consumption of sugar in the form of ice cream, soft drinks, and candy. The following incident had remarkable implications.

In 1949, Dr. Sandler spoke on the radio in Asheville, North Carolina and warned that parents feed their children no sugar or foods containing sugar in an effort to avert a polio outbreak. He also recommended a high protein diet with low starch vegetables as being the best protection against low blood sugar, a condition making people susceptible to polio. The typical "polio profile" was heavy physical exertion coupled with high consumption of refined carbohydrates. [209, 210]

The people responded and store sales of sugar, candy, ice cream, cakes, soft drinks, etc. dropped sharply and remained at low levels for the rest of the summer. One southern producer of ice cream shipped one million fewer gallons of ice cream than usual, during the first week following the release of the diet story. Polio in North Carolina was 2,402 cases in 1948. In 1949, after Dr. Sandler's publicity, there were 214 cases! The country as a whole showed an *increase* in the number of cases from 1948 to 1949. This was accomplished *without* a vaccine. These remarkable results were widely reported on the radio and in the newspapers before the vaccine was invented. [211]

The Decline of Polio

Polio was on the decline *before* vaccines were invented or widespread. Where the vaccine was not so extensively used in Europe, epidemics *also* ended. This suggests that the low incidence of polio in the 1960's and 1970's is a reflection of the low point in the natural cycle of polio epidemics. [211]

In Australia, as with other countries, the dramatic decline in polio occurred even prior to the invention of the vaccine in 1955. [213] The incidence of death from polio in Great Britain peaked in 1950 and had declined 82% before 1956 when the vaccine was first introduced. [214] Finland seemed to have wiped out polio when only a fraction of its population had been vaccinated. [215] In light of these facts, one could easily assume polio was on a natural decline before vaccines and the decrease and disappearance was just a natural waning of the disease. Some experts have concluded that the polio vaccine does not deserve credit for the disappearance of polio. Because so many other diseases have come and gone without the use of vaccines, this seems a legitimate posture.

In a time of epidemics, fear of polio ran high and faith in medicine was held as "the only hope." Ironically, it is even possible that the fear of polio was actually *fueled* by the creation of a vaccine. It would have been unconscionable to let a declining disease die out on its own when it was believed that a "cure" for a dreaded crippler existed. Even today, parents seem to have more fear of those diseases for which there is a vaccine.

Questionable Reporting of Polio

Dr. Bernard Greenberg, head of the Department of Biostatistics of the University of North Carolina School of Public Health, testified during the 1962 Congressional Hearings on HR 10541. He said that polio increased substantially from 1957 to 1958 (50%) and from 1958 to 1959 (80%) *after* the introduction of mass immunization programs that were often compulsory, but statistics were manipulated and statements made by the Public Health Service gave the opposite impression. [216]

These are some of the specific ways polio statistics were manipulated:

- Redefinition of an epidemic requiring more cases in order to be classified as an epidemic. Before the Salk vaccine: 20 cases per 100,000. After the Salk vaccine: 35 cases per 100,000 per year. [Polio could enter non-epidemic proportions sooner, making it appear as though the vaccine reduced the number of cases.]

- Redefinition of the disease so a patient had to exhibit paralytic symptoms for at least 60 days after onset of polio. Prior to 1954, the patient had to exhibit paralytic symptoms for only 24 hours. [Fewer cases of polio, by definition, are reported after 1954.]

- Large numbers of cases of Cocksackie virus and aseptic meningitis were mislabeled as paralytic polio. Prior to July 1, 1958, these cases were reported as non-paralytic polio but are now reported as viral or aseptic meningitis. [217] [Fewer cases of polio reported after 1958.]

What would be considered a polio case one year, would not be considered polio another year. This would show a reduction in polio cases exclusively by virtue of reporting methods. Therefore, credit for a "declining" disease is given to the vaccine, when a great number of polio cases did not get recorded.

If one assumes polio was on a decline before the vaccine and then headed back up after the vaccine, then the vaccine could have actually *interfered* with polio's inevitable natural decline.

The Polio Vaccine

The first vaccine for polio to be introduced was from a killed virus and was injected. This vaccine is still used on rare occasions. Now (since 1961) children are given four oral doses of the live virus vaccine before the age of seven. The "live oral trivalent" polio vaccine is a mixture of three types of attenuated polio viruses which have been propagated in monkey kidney tissue. [218]

The killed virus vaccine was abandoned in favor of the live oral vaccine because it was thought to be more effective, carrying fewer side effects. Many people are unaware today, that in the 50's and early 60's, there was ongoing debate over which vaccine was better and whether which actually caused or prevented polio. Concern about the vaccines actually causing polio made *many* people choose not to vaccinate for fear of catching polio. News of this debate has long since disappeared and the contemporary populace is coaxed into believing that in the early days of the polio vaccine that there was universal acceptance.

The Polio Vaccine Reactions and Failures

The polio vaccine's primary reaction is that it can directly cause polio. The polio vaccine "fails" because if it can *cause* polio it fails to prevent polio. So the polio vaccine reactions and failures are not distinguished in most discussions.

Damage suits during the 1950's gave indisputable proof that it was the Salk and Sabin vaccines that caused numerous cases of paralysis and death in addition to many cases of post-vaccinal encephalitis. [219]

In 1976, Dr. Jonas Salk, creator of the killed virus vaccine testified that the live virus vaccine, created by Dr. Albert Sabin, was the principal if not the sole cause of the 140 polio cases reported in the United States since 1961, and is riskier than no vaccine at all. [220] Even the Salk vaccine has been shown to cause tumors in experimental animals. [221] Confirmed cases of vaccine-associated paralytic polio have occurred in many countries since 1961 when the oral vaccine was introduced. [222]

- Of the 119 cases of polio occurring in the United States between 1969 and 1976, 55 clearly followed vaccination of an individual or a close contact. [223]

- Of the 18 cases of polio in 1977, three cases occurred in recent vaccine recipients, and ten had been in close contact with recently vaccinated people. [224]

- In California during 1979 and 1980, all reported cases of polio were acquired in other countries or were suspiciously associated with the vaccine. [225]

- Of the 21 cases of paralytic polio which occurred in this country in 1982 and 1983, all were vaccine-related. [226]

- From 1980 to 1985, 55 cases of paralytic polio were reported. Of these cases, 51 were caused by the vaccine and four occurred in people returning from developing countries. [227]

Reported in the United States each year are six to eight adult cases of polio after close contact with recently vaccinated children. [228] The risk of acquiring polio from this vaccine is one in 560,000 for the first dose. The risk to household contacts is about one in 6,000,000 vaccine recipients and one in 23,000,000 for community contacts. The risk of acquiring wild polio in this country is *zero.* [229]

There is no chance of getting polio naturally but there is a chance of getting polio from the vaccine, either directly or indirectly. A common way that polio is contracted from a child who has been vaccinated is by contact with diapers. The polio virus is excreted through the stool and urine for four to six weeks after the vaccine has been given. [230]

Apparently the attenuated virus used in the vaccine occasionally mutates during multiplication in the intestines and become virulent again. [231] Cases of paralysis and death have occurred in family members of recently vaccinated babies. The medical reasoning is that other "susceptible" family members should also be vaccinated. There is a *greater* chance of "catching" polio *directly* from the vaccine than there is from a *contact* with a person receiving a vaccine. So, it is illogical to assume that the very agent that can cause polio can "protect" other members of society from possible vaccine-associated polio.

Today, reducing polio cases in this country is as easy as eliminating vaccinating for it. One could therefore extrapolate that the polio vaccine actually interfered with the reduction in an epidemic while it was causing more cases than would naturally occur. In the early days of the polio vaccine, when such a relatively large portion of the population was susceptible to the polio virus (in the 50's) then it would be easy to assume many more cases of polio were vaccine-related.

Polio vaccination is fueled by the fear of polio from the 1950's and by the *assumption* that it prevented polio even though statistics suggest otherwise.

To Sum It Up

☐ The rate of polio was declining before the vaccine was introduced. Polio waned in other countries, without the vaccines, as fast or faster than in the United States.

☐ Questionable methods of reporting attributed to lowering the polio case count. This alone could have reduced "epidemics" significantly.

☐ There was much debate over which vaccine (killed or live) was better in the early days of polio vaccination. Many chose neither for fear of getting polio from the vaccine. The history of this debate has been removed from modern questions about the polio vaccine.

☐ All cases of polio in the U.S. are directly related to the polio vaccine. There is a higher chance of getting polio from the vaccine than from contact with a recipient of the polio vaccine.

☐ With no polio in this country and with the vaccine being the only cause, there is little justification to vaccinate.

☐ There are experts who believe that the vaccine is not responsible for the disappearance of polio.

MENINGITIS

The Disease

There are between 8,000 and 15,000 cases of Haemophilus influenzae type b meningitis (Hib meningitis) per year in the United States. Hib meningitis death rate is 3% to 8% of cases. Children under 6 months of age are protected by maternal antibodies, and breastfeeding reduces cases of meningitis. Hib meningitis occurs most often in children 6 to 7 months of age. The rate decreases rapidly with increasing age. [232] Haemophilus influenzae is found in the throats of 30% of healthy, normal people, without ever showing symptoms of the disease. [233] One could assume natural immunities are already protecting people to a large degree without ever having vaccinated the entire population.

The Hib Vaccine

There are several meningitis vaccines licensed for general use in the United States. They are of two types: the polysaccharide and the conjugate. Generally the polysaccharide vaccine (licensed in 1985) is used on children 24 months or older, and the conjugate is used on children 18 months or older. Ongoing clinical trials are investigating the efficacy of using the conjugate vaccine in babies as young as 2 months old with subsequent boosters. [234]

(Latest Update: On October 4, 1990, the FDA approved the HibTITER for use on babies at 2, 4 and 6 months plus a fourth booster at 15 months. The vaccine can be given at the same time as the DPT. This vaccine was previously approved in 1988 for use in children 15 months or older. [235] It is interesting to note that as recently as April 1990, an article appeared in *Pediatrics* that showed confidence had not yet been gained that Hib vaccine could be effective in infants. See quote, this chapter.)

In a conjugate vaccine, the polysaccharide of the bacterial capsule is coupled with some type of protein carrier, such as tetanus toxoid, diphtheria toxoid, a variant of diphtheria toxin and a carrier that employs the outer membrane protein of Neisseria meningitis. [236]

The Hib Vaccine Reactions

Polysaccharide:

A study of 152 reports of vaccine reactions submitted to the FDA, 1985 to 1986:

Convulsions (with and without fever); anaphylactoid allergic reactions; serum sickness-like reactions (joint pain, rashes, and edema); one death within 4 hours of vaccination; 63 reports of proven H influenzae type b that occurred soon after immunization [237] [these were considered "failures" but if the vaccine caused the disease it would be considered a reaction].

Conjugate:

High fevers; erythema, swelling/induration; irritability; drowsiness; diarrhea/nausea/vomiting; respiratory symptoms; rash [238]

The Hib Vaccine Failures

Polysaccharide:

The Haemophilus b polysaccharide vaccine was licensed in the United States in April 1985. In randomized clinical trials in Finland, the vaccine had no effect in preventing the disease in children younger than 18 months old. Therefore, the American Academy of Pediatrics recommended vaccination for all children 24 to 59 months of age. In addition, the Immunization Practices Advisory Committee (ACIP) of the U.S. Public Health Service recommended the vaccine for children 18 months or older who were at increased risk of disease such as children attending day care. [239] A study in Minnesota in August 1985:

- Of the 88 cases of Hib, 36 (41%) occurred in vaccinated children.

- The vaccine's protective efficacy was determined to be between negative 55% and negative 58% [-55%, -58%]. [240]

In spite of studies having "adjusted their findings due to the child's attendance in day care" and in one instance those who got meningitis within three weeks of the vaccine were thrown out of the study, the protective efficacy was less than expected before licensure. Several studies showed numbers such as -55%, -29%, 31% 41%, 71% up to 92% effective in "preventing" meningitis. [241]

In addition to the failure to prevent Hib meningitis and the known reactions and death, there are two studies to confirm that *Hib meningitis occurs greater than six times more often in children vaccinated with the Hib vaccine.* Among 16 cases of Hib occurring within 14 days of vaccination reported to the FDA, 10 were clustered within the first 72 hours. [242]

Doubtful that the vaccine is preventing Hib at all, studies tend to show it actually increases the likelihood of a child getting Hib meningitis.

Conjugate:

"However, it is clear that much remains to be learned about

the nuances of the immune responses to the different conjugate vaccines and that not all populations at increased risk for disease caused by H influenzae type b necessarily will be protected by all of the conjugate vaccines currently available or under investigation." [243]

To Sum It Up

☐ There are serious side effects associated with the vaccines.

☐ Children younger than 18 months of age are at a higher risk of contracting Hib meningitis but the vaccines are deemed "effective" only in older children.

☐ Ongoing clinical trials have not yet "proven" that Hib meningitis can be prevented in infants or in children older than 18 months.

☐ There is strong evidence that suggests that the Hib vaccine actually *increases* the likelihood of contracting Hib meningitis.

CHICKEN POX (Varicella)

The Disease

In normal children, the risk of death from complications of chicken pox is 0.0014%. Children who are cancer and leukemia patients undergoing chemotherapy and those with inborn immune deficiencies are more likely to develop complications from chicken pox. Adults who contract chicken pox generally have a longer and more serious illness. In adults, the complication rate is higher than in children. [244]

Varicella-zoster virus can be stored in nerve cells after natural chicken pox infection. This can cause a recurrence of infection later in life. The subsequent infection is known as herpes zoster or shingles, a very painful skin eruption that may last for several weeks. [245]

While chicken pox is uncomfortable, it is not generally a dangerous disease in children. Parents would not wish it on their children, but they do not have any unreasonable fears of this disease.

The Chicken Pox Vaccine

Though the vaccine was developed in 1973, it is not approved for widespread use among normal children. It is currently used only in children with cancer and leukemia. Ongoing studies are determining proper dosage, reactions and effectiveness in normal children. Evaluation of using the vaccine in combination with the measles, mumps and rubella vaccine will probably lead to replacement of the MMR with the MMRV. [246]

The Chicken Pox Vaccine Reactions

Some experts feel that if a vaccine were to be widely used, we would see increases in Reyes syndrome, which can result in brain damage or death. Unusual cases of varicella-zoster illness may also occur, as unusual cases of measles and mumps occur after those vaccines. The most common reaction has been a generalized rash that resembles naturally acquired chicken pox. At least 5% to 10% of the vaccine recipients acquire this eruption. [247]

Varicella vaccine has caused zoster in normal children. [248] Varicella zoster virus may also be a cause of cancer. Varicella-zoster-infected human cells have transformed mouse cells to cancerous cells in a laboratory. [249] There is also concern that the vaccine may have a role in causing shingles later in life.

The Chicken Pox Vaccine Failures

In studies of vaccinated children with leukemia, 2% to 10% of their siblings developed varicella vaccine virus eruptions. So, the eruptions caused by the vaccine can be spread to others. [250] Therefore, if the vaccine can cause chicken pox it fails to prevent chicken pox at least some of the time.

Dr. Philip Brunell describes a reluctance to use the vaccine in normal children because "chicken pox, which is relatively mild in childhood, might increase in frequency during adult life when it is much more severe." [251] Another warning: If immunity wanes, one would not want to vaccinate against varicella routinely in childhood because of the possibility of creating a population of varicella-susceptible adults. [252] This would not be improving society's overall health because complications of chicken pox in *adults* can be worse than from measles or mumps.

To Sum It Up

☐ Chicken pox is a mild disease in childhood.

☐ Vaccinating for chicken pox could actually increase cases in adolescence and adulthood.

☐ The varicella-zoster virus is stored in the nerve cells and can cause recurrent infections of herpes zoster or shingles.

☐ Chicken pox that has been caused by a vaccine can spread to others.

☐ The chicken pox vaccine has not been approved for wide-spread use by normal children. Once the vaccine is approved it is likely that the life-time effects will not be known until a life-time has passed.

PNEUMONIA

The Disease

Streptococcus pneumonia is a bacterium associated with many cases of pneumonia, meningitis, bacteremia (systemic infection in the blood stream) and ear infections. The bacterium's increasing resistance to antibiotics has stimulated vaccine research.

The Pneumococcal Vaccine

Only those children at increased risk of serious pneumonococcal infections are receiving this vaccine. These include children with certain chronic diseases that impair the immune system and those who have had their spleen removed. [253]

In 1977 a pneumococcal vaccine was licensed containing 14 types of S pneumonia. In 1983, it was replaced by a vaccine with 23 types. Because of their limited success the new vaccine technology has taken the polysaccharide vaccine and bonded it to a protein carrier to produce a conjugate vaccine that researchers hope will be more "successful." [254]

This pneumococcal vaccine will be made available soon to all children. It will be deemed "safe and effective" in preventing pneumonia, meningitis, and ear infections. It will probably be combined with other existing vaccines as part of the recommended immunization schedule. This would follow the course of the Hib vaccine which is accepted and widely used in spite of its very poor history of preventing meningitis. [255]

The Pneumococcal Vaccine Reactions

Approximately 50% develop swelling and pain at the injection site. Other possible reactions include: muscle pain, severe swelling, high fevers and severe allergic reactions. [256]

The Pneumococcal Vaccine Failures

Four studies found little or no effect in the vaccine's ability to prevent pneumococcal infections. The currently licensed polysaccharide vaccine is ineffective in children under 2 years old. [257]

To Sum It Up

☐ The pneumococcal vaccine can cause severe reactions.

☐ Its ability to prevent pneumococcal infections has been questioned and remains unproven.

AIDS AND VACCINES

• **The Disease**

• **The Vaccine Link**

• **The Spread of AIDS**

• **AIDS and Politics**

Why a chapter on AIDS in a book about childhood vaccines? The fact that AIDS *could have* been caused, spread, or aggravated by the small pox vaccine makes it a vaccine issue. The fact that AIDS victims could be "creating" other epidemics of infectious diseases, given their lack of an immune system, thereby spawning further vaccine research, makes it a vaccine issue. The fact that scientists are seriously considering the possibility of developing an AIDS vaccine, which might prove to be the most fatal fiasco in vaccine history, makes it a vaccine issue.

Fear of this contemporary dreaded epidemic will only increase as death rates soar exponentially in the next few years. There will be a fervent call for medicine to "do something" and that something is already pointing to a vaccine.

The Disease

The AIDS virus seems to be harbored in the T-lymphocyte

system of the immune system. The "helper" and the "suppressor" cells are the two main mechanisms. The ratio of T4 (helper cells) to T8 (suppressor cells) in a healthy individual is normally 2:1. In AIDS victims, this ratio is reversed. (This ratio has also been shown to be temporarily reversed after a tetanus booster shot.) Reversal in the ratio means the suppressor cells which, under normal conditions prevent the T-lymphocyte system from producing when not needed, are now suppressing the immune system when needed most. This allows other infectious organisms known as "opportunistic infections" to take hold and multiply. [258]

Those infected with the AIDS virus frequently carry, cannot be cured of, and are highly infectious for tuberculosis, cytomegalovirus (CMV), salmonella, herpes, and toxoplasmosis. There is currently a tuberculosis epidemic in the United States that has been directly attributed to AIDS. An incurable form of tuberculosis has been found in up to 50% of AIDS patients on autopsy. Tuberculosis can infect young, healthy people without any immunodeficiency and has been shown to have contaminated hospital water supplies where high numbers of AIDS patients are treated. AIDS victims also have a 20 fold increase in the incidence of salmonella, which has also assumed epidemic proportions in the U.S. [259]

The Vaccine Link

On May 11, 1987 the *London Times* front page reported that the World Health Organization (WHO) "triggered" the AIDS epidemic in Africa through the small pox immunization program. The geographical sites chosen in 1972 for small pox eradication (Uganda and other African states, Haiti and Brazil) coincided with the recent past of AIDS epidemiology. Where the most concentrated effort of small pox "eradication" took place are exactly the areas of the largest incidence of AIDS. This information was never printed in any major American daily paper, nor did radio or television news cover this report. [260]

It is possible the small pox vaccine carried the AIDS virus. It is also possible that it triggered previous carriers of HIV. This could explain why AIDS is spread more evenly between males and females and children in Africa and Brazil than in the West. [261] The spread of AIDS in the United States could very easily be explained by an experimental hepatitis vaccine used exclusively on promiscuous male homosexuals between the ages of 20 and 40 in New York in 1978 and in San Francisco and Los Angeles in 1980. [262]

The Spread of AIDS

There are methods of transmitting AIDS that are not well publicized for fear of causing public panic. But AIDS does not confine itself to high risk groups. Much documentation shows AIDS in health-care workers, lab technicians and siblings. Their only known risk was casual contact with a known AIDS patient. [263]

Health-care workers, lab technicians and dentists are advised to use masks, gloves and gowns and thoroughly disinfect after treating AIDS patients, yet the public is led to believe AIDS cannot be transmitted through casual contact.

Contrary to medical dogma, condoms are not safety against the spread of AIDS. The failure rate of preventing pregnancy with condoms is as high as 10%. [264] Also, the pores in the rubber of a condom are bigger than the AIDS virus itself. [265] Condom studies done with spouses showed that 3 out of 10 were infected in spite of condom use. [266]

AIDS can be spread through the nation's blood supply. In a study done in 1986, 20,000 blood donors repeatedly reacted positively to one test for AIDS (Elisa) but negatively to another test (Western Blot). [267] A person can incubate the AIDS virus up to 34 months before enough antibodies in his blood could be detected by a test, meanwhile he could still transmit the virus. And there continues to be new strains of the virus for which there is no test. [268] Screening for AIDS in the blood supply has improved, however it doesn't change the fact that a person can have AIDS long before it can be detected in their blood, thereby reaching the blood supply.

Some products derived from the blood supply include: insect venom therapy (for allergies), gamma globulin, RhoGAM, antihemophilic globulin, hepatitis vaccine, organ transplants and tetanus immune globulin. [269, 270]

A Possible AIDS Vaccine?

Finding a vaccine or cure for AIDS is probably next to impossible. The virus actually integrates its own DNA into the cells of humans. Therefore, when cells are reproduced, the AIDS virus is also reproduced. Curing AIDS has been compared to the ability to cure the common cold and all genetic defects, and being able to change the color of a person's eyes. Its rate of mutation is 5 times greater than any known virus (there are 75 different types already), and the same person can harbor multiple forms of the virus. [271] Potential manufacturers are extremely concerned about liability. [272] AIDS is an RNA virus and no one has ever made a vaccine against an RNA virus before. [273] California was under pressure from potential manufacturers of an AIDS vaccine in order to formulate policy on compensating victims who are damaged by a new vaccine so a special task force was formed.

Hope for a vaccine is encouraged while blatantly ignoring the near impossibility of this task. Because people can have AIDS for years and years before any signs or symptoms become evident, a new vaccine could not be deemed "safe" for at least a generation.

AIDS and Politics

If one believes that AIDS is exclusively a sexually transmitted disease, there should be concern because it is not treated as other diseases of this type. With AIDS, previous sexual contacts are not traced. It is illegal for a doctor to tell a spouse that he is married to someone with AIDS. Further, testing done anonymously has allowed patients, who do not know they have AIDS, to circulate freely. [274]

Controversy on the origins of AIDS and how it is spread are not given proper treatment in the media. Never before in history has an epidemic been treated with such bias and disregard for public health. Existing laws regarding public health are altered or ignored when it comes to AIDS. It has become purely a political and social issue rather than simply a public health threat.

HOMEOPATHY

This chapter is included because many readers have asked for information on homeopathic vaccines It is a brief explanation of a possible alternative to traditional vaccines, since some parents have a strong need to find a substitute. There is a homeopathic "vaccine" for every childhood disease for which there is a traditional vaccine, plus scarlet fever and influenza. [275] They are manufactured from humans with the disease. No animal products are ever used. Unlike traditional vaccines, they are derived from humans, highly diluted, given orally and based on individual requirements.

But disagreement exists among homeopathic practitioners about the safety and validity of introducing a homeopathic medication into the body if there are no existing symptoms. Usually, homeopathic medicines are prescribed on the basis of symptom expression. [276, 277]

Although far less invasive and far less risky than traditional vaccines, the question still remains whether homeopathic vaccines can actually prevent those diseases. And do homeopathic vaccines go contrary to its own principles of addressing symptoms while eliciting the help of the body's own immune system? These questions need to be reconciled before proceeding with the homeopathic alternative.

Some homeopathic practitioners feel more comfortable when a child undergoes a "constitutional" homeopathic treatment in order to prevent disease in general. There also has been reported success in reversing vaccine reactions or damage by using homeopathic remedies.

Part III

The Heart of the Vaccine Issue

VACCINATION PERPETUATION

- **Parents, Fear, Anxiety and Guilt**
- **Denial**
- **Exposing the Vaccine Philosophy**

Parents, Fear, Anxiety and Guilt

Since most vaccines are directed specifically at babies and children, assumptions and theories are perpetuated while the vaccine philosophy feeds off the emotions of the uninformed and fearful parents. No one wants to deny the best for their children, so vaccination establishes an easy avenue that leads to accepting traditional medicine in the form of artificial immunization.

The perception, that there is no control over diseases and that they attack at random, increases fear. With more profound understanding of how diseases operate and what can be done to prevent them, fear of disease decreases. With less fear the "reasons" for vaccinating become less significant. Fifty-thousand people die in car accidents every year but most do not live in constant fear that they will "catch" an accident. They overtly control the situation; they can drive defensively and soberly, maintain the brakes in the car, keep the tires in good condition, etc. Somehow, because of their role in the prevention of accidents, they tend not to fear them in the same way. We should be more afraid of how and when we make ourselves *susceptible* to disease, than of the disease itself.

If vaccines did not exist, fear of disease would be *less*, not more. Promoting vaccines and promoting fear go hand-in-hand. This effect is proven by the fact that parents tend to be *more* fearful of diseases for which there is a vaccine than afraid of much more pervasive or dangerous diseases for which there is *no* vaccine. They are told they are "taking chances" when they choose not to vaccinate. But if there were no vaccines, they wouldn't be "taking chances" any more than they would be with car accidents or cancer or tuberculosis. Also, many parents are amazed upon finding out diseases that are so mild these days are still vaccinated against. They thought they were *supposed* to be afraid of them because there *is* a vaccine against them.

It's natural for parents to have a certain degree of anxiety over the possibility of illness in their child. It is this anxiety over diseases that gets all the attention, and the anxiety over vaccine damage is underplayed. Because of pressure and fear tactics, parents can easily feel guilty for questioning vaccine procedures or for even considering the idea of not vaccinating their child. Parents find that this kind of guilt can be temporarily relieved by giving-in to the vaccine philosophy. The parents can feel, that in spite of everything else, at least they did their "duty."

When a parent chooses not to vaccinate, he too must overcome the same guilt that is imposed on him by society. It is perceived that vaccines are a proven method of preventing diseases. It is almost unheard-of that anyone could possibly reject such a "gift." So, by not vaccinating, a person must turn his back on a whole system that is very much a part of his culture and society. This separation can cause overwhelming feelings of guilt for going against the status-quo. No one usually considers that a non-vaccinated child was possibly protected from vaccine damage. Imagine the *real* guilt of a parent whose child suffered as a result of an action that was planned, calculated and not an accident or left to chance. The self-reproach can be tremendous. When vaccine damage occurs, it is perceived that the act of vaccinating could have been withheld, therefore parents feel they could have taken an active role in preventing a damaging situation for their child.

Epidemics are usually classified in the "natural disaster" category—an "act of God." When a thousand people perish in a flood, tornado or earthquake, it is a social tragedy. But that grief is felt much differently than the sorrow and grief after the brutal murder of a member of the community. There is public outrage. There is combined hope for expedient capture and prosecution of the criminal. The whole community is affected with anger and disgust. This is just one death, not one thousand. Similarly, when an "act of God" claims a victim of a disease, it is felt differently than the outrage felt after vaccine-injury or vaccine-death. Many parents find comfort in knowing that above all else, they were not responsible for *purposely* subjecting their child to the risk that the vaccine could injure.

Only because "science" has given a choice (to choose a form of technology or reject it), does anxiety exist. Anxiety over making a decision results in contemplating the idea that a person would be left guilty if not making the right choice. Natural anxieties and guilt play right into the vaccine philosophy.

Denial

A mother's son died 33 hours after the DPT shot. She confronted her pediatrician only to be met with denials. The coroner also tried to deny any connection, writing on the death certificate "death due to irreversible shock." He said he "couldn't write down on the death certificate that he died from a DPT reaction because the state's standing on immunizations would be in an uproar." [278]

Medical professionals have often stated that broadcasting side effects of vaccines to the public would cause unnecessary concern among parents and hinder the vaccine campaign. [279]

Motivated to continue selling vaccines, and in order to prevent scaring the public away, study results are often manipulated or not publicized. For example, 63 reports of Hib that occurred soon after the immunization were considered vaccine "failures." This means that the vaccine failed to protect against Hib. In other words, the child would have gotten Hib *anyway* at exactly the same time. These probably *should* have been reported as reactions, at the very least, because a case could be made that the vaccine *caused* Hib meningitis. [280]

The Small Pox Vaccine Gives Historical Perspective

- Prior to small pox vaccination in England, the highest death rate for any two year period from small pox was 2,000. Two years *after* the compulsory enforcement of the vaccine (during 1870-1871), 23,062 people had died of small pox. Did the vaccine cause the increase, or was it a coincidence?

- In Germany, 124, 948 people died, all were vaccinated.

- In Bavaria, 29,000 cases with 3,994 deaths; all were vaccinated.

- In Japan, 165, 774 cases with 28, 979 deaths between 1886 and 1892; vaccinations were compulsory.

- Every Filipino was vaccinated one to six times during 1879-1919. Twelve years after the introduction of compulsory vaccinations there were 71, 450 deaths from small pox. Prior to the introduction of compulsory vaccinations in the Philippines, the death rate for small pox was 10%. After the compulsory vaccine laws were introduced, the death rate from small pox was 75%.

- In Australia there were no vaccination laws. There were 3 cases of small pox in 15 years. [281]

The trick wasn't surviving small pox, it was surviving the vaccine! But these are certainly considered "coincidence" and not cause. Otherwise, why did they continue after such obvious "failures?" Small pox was continued worldwide for 30 years in spite of the fact that the vaccine was virtually the only source of the disease. Yet, the small pox vaccine is unanimously given credit for wiping out a dreaded disease.

The same is happening with the polio vaccine in the United States. The polio vaccine is virtually the only source of that disease.

Whenever a casual observer might say that vaccines *caused* certain results, the studies conclude they are coincidence. Sudden Infant Death Syndrome following a DPT vaccine is *almost always* considered temporal, or a timely coincidence. In other words, the baby would have died anyway. With these kinds of "scientific" studies, it would be just as easy (and perhaps more accurate) to say that the vaccine could have caused these results than automatically assuming coincidence.

Conclusions such as "coincidence" are arrived at due to a faulty hypothesis. Most studies begin with the hypothesis that vaccines are safe and they work. If studies were begun with the hypothesis that vaccines are inherently dangerous and probably don't work, the conclusions would be entirely different, based on the *same* results, using the *same* statistics. The facts and figures would back up this finding as easily as the "coincidence" finding.

When declining diseases were coupled with the introduction of vaccines, it was *easy* to attribute this result to the effectiveness of the vaccines. This was concluded *even though* all other diseases, for which there was no vaccine also declined. Again, one could easily draw the conclusion that vaccines had nothing to do with it. According to the *World Health Statistics Annual 1973-1976, Volume 2*, there has been a steady decline of infectious diseases in most developing countries regardless of the percentage of vaccines administered. Researchers pointed out that infectious diseases disappeared as the result of sanitation, improved public water supplies, improved personal hygiene and better distribution and increased consumption of fresh fruits and vegetables.[282]

The World Health Organization has conceded that the best vaccine against common infectious diseases is an adequate diet. Despite this, they made it perfectly clear that they still intend to promote mass immunization campaigns. In the 1940's Dr. Sandler successfully averted a polio outbreak in his community by recommending parents refrain from giving their children sugar and starches. Sales of sugar and sugar-containing products plummeted, and when other parts of the country saw huge increases in polio, his area showed a *decrease* (see polio chapter). This "experiment" was probably never repeated. Money was lost in sugar sales. Could there have been pressure from business? Was it not politically wise to advertise the restricted use of these products that so many relied upon for income? Where are the priorities?

Doctors have the most to gain by current vaccination laws. They are responsible in part for pushing the idea of "no shots, no school." Vaccines, after all, are what drives healthy children into doctor's offices when they might not otherwise have reason to be there.

As recommended by the vaccine manufacturers and other officials, vaccines are not to be given to children with acute illnesses. But in practice, vaccines are routinely administered to children with little consideration of the child's current health conditions. A child going into a vaccination clinic who is "behind" in the vaccination schedule runs the risk of having two or three doses, *at the same time.* This is unheard-of in the accepted vaccination practices. They go against their own requirements and their own rules in a non-scientific and non-caring way. Is this denial of safe medical practice? What are the motivations? Political? Economic?

Very often a doctor refuses to culture (in order to confirm a diagnosis of pertussis) if the child had been previously vaccinated for pertussis, and then has no hesitation in an unvaccinated child. This shows a refusal to discover the truth. Is he afraid of finding out the vaccine didn't work? Does he want to "prove" the other child should have been vaccinated? Is he afraid of too much negative publicity? *This happens all the time.* Where is the concern for truth and improving health? Can health only be accomplished through *one* approved method? When evidence points negatively at vaccines, the accuser is assumed wrong, not the vaccines.

If medical science were "up front" with the public, they would not cover up mistakes, or explain them away. They would advertise both sides of the vaccine philosophy. They would admit to the impossibility of doing scientific double blind tests on a population. Basically, they would not be so quick to deny any information that might threaten a neat little package called "vaccination."

These kinds of denial perpetuate vaccine practices. If one believes that vaccines work and are relatively harmless, then he will not and will *never* see them as the cause of something negative, as long as he can excuse and explain away the inconsistencies and *make* his findings fit his hypothesis. The incidence of Hib meningitis has increased over the past three decades. Some observers associate this increase with the administration of other vaccines and their apparent ability to impair immune system resistance. So, we could be creating a situation where instead of getting to the root cause of disease (impairment of the immune system) we create yet another vaccine (Hib) to "cure" the problem. We could very well be creating vaccines to deal with a problem that vaccines created! All from stubbornly sticking to the hypothesis that vaccines are safe and that they work.

Making someone a little bit sick to possibly prevent an illness sometime in the future is contrary to medicine's true purpose: to prevent and/or cure diseases. This involves finding cause and ways of maintaining health. As long as you assume that a disease is "taken care of" by a vaccine, you close the door to prevention, because in essence you've made everyone "a little bit sick" and you close the door to finding cause, because by accepting vaccination, the true cause of disease is no longer relevant.

Exposing the Vaccine Philosophy

Everyday, the media, doctors, and health departments advertise that vaccines work and that they are safe. It is probably the biggest untruth ever forced on the public. But this could not have been so successful if the people were not eager to believe, at all costs.

Vaccine manufacturers will not stand behind their products unless forced to do so in court. Other manufacturers do not have this luxury. Products are recalled on the basis of their possible hazards (cars, for example). But vaccines enjoy a kind of insulation from this usual product responsibility.

"Shots" in our society have become so common-place and so accepted that it pervades children's literature and school curriculum, making the doubter feel out of place and in another world. A child afraid of doctors is taken as perfectly normal. When an unvaccinated child goes to a doctor for injuries or other reasons, everyone is so amazed at the child's acceptance of these medical people. The child's experience has never been awful so they don't take these strangers as enemies. Why are most children afraid? Because they remember the shots and then society says, "Oh, it's normal."

Vaccines are here to stay as long as people accept what is not normal as normal. Because it happens all the time, does not make it normal.

- Doctors "use" vaccines as a way to feel they have an active role in eliminating disease.

- Schools "use" vaccines as a way to maintain safety on school grounds. Public safety goes a long way, politically.

- In-laws, etc. "use" them to be sure that inexperienced parents are giving a child the "best" care possible.

- Parents "use" them to relieve guilt of not being perfect parents and/or relieve any perceived future guilt that might be due to the child's becoming sick.

We all have found ways to "use" vaccines and giving them up will not come easy. It would require looking at life, economics, politics and how we care for our children, entirely differently. A tall order and not likely to happen on a wide scale in our or our child's lifetime. But parents everywhere are taking back responsibility for their child's health. Their reliance has shifted to good diet, clean living and low stress environment.

Exposing the vaccine philosophy has zeroed-in on questionable scientific practices, public suppression of negative aspects of vaccines, scare tactics used by medical authorities on vulnerable parents, cover ups and denials of pointed scientific findings. This could read like an international spy novel, except the tragedy is, it's true.

The vaccine philosophy regularly transcends logical thinking. Using societal pressures and cultural conditioning as forces to mold behavior, the belief systems in a culture get so deeply ingrained that people can act outside common sense and inner direction.

People believe that vaccination is the panacea of disease, and this leads to quick acceptance of the vaccine philosophy. The vaccine philosophy contends that diseases must be eliminated, wiped-out. But disease will not be conquered. *Health must be maintained and then disease is absent.* Instead of seeking ways to maintain health and improve living conditions, the heavy responsibility is entirely turned over to physicians, drugs and government.

Parents operate with a strong motivation to do "everything possible" for their children. Because they cannot live the child's life twice, once with vaccines and once without, they are forced to make a decision according to their *beliefs*, because with vaccination, the possibility of the child getting that disease still remains.

Vaccination takes a pre-determined course of action that is to single out certain diseases and find a "cure" in a dubious form of "prevention." Then it is thought that the "battle" of one disease is won. But the "war" of finding *true* health goes on. If a person were to step on a piece of glass, he may then spend the rest of his time looking for glass and in his preoccupation, he might run into a wall. So, using this analogy, we focus on "protecting against one disease" but may be running into "walls" when it comes to the total health of an individual. There are many would-be vaccines on the horizon.

There is talk of bringing back a more "effective" killed polio vaccine; giving measles boosters; giving several doses and/or several combinations of vaccines in a single doctor's visit, and on and on. Certainly, vaccines and vaccine practices will change. But will that be better, or just a different verse of the same song? As long as the *philosophy* is the same, the testing and study results will be questionable.

The vaccine philosophy is trapped in a very narrow perspective. There are many more diseases than there are vaccines to "prevent" them. Shouldn't we concentrate on finding ways to improve general health, rather than singling out each disease? Taking the vaccine philosophy to the extreme, a baby would receive 100 vaccines on his birth date to "protect" him from all possible infections. Would the child ever be predisposed to these diseases anyway? Could he possibly survive that kind of inoculation? Of course not. But to take something to the extreme serves to show the absurdity of heading toward more vaccines instead of less.

Now that we have vaccines for numerous diseases, and more to come, great assumptions are made and the history of a given disease is recorded only with relationship to the vaccine. This is an example of the mental gymnastics required in order to keep alive the vaccine philosophy and perpetuate all present and future vaccines:

Let's take a hypothetical "vaccine" of pure sterile water. If the "disease" declines, credit is given to the vaccine. If the disease spreads, it would be held that not enough people are getting the vaccine and consequently stricter compulsory vaccination laws would be enforced. If "vaccinated" people get the disease, then increased doses would be recommended. If the disease disappears, it would be recommended that vaccination continue, to keep it away. If other diseases occur, new vaccines will be developed. No matter what the results of vaccination, the rigid mind-set remains unchanged: vaccines will always be safe and good and they work.

SUMMARY

Vaccines *seem* to work because of the current near lack of these childhood diseases. But even in epidemic circumstances it has never been proven that vaccination can be responsible for reducing the spread of disease. Without sound scientific principles, vaccination is an act performed in desperate *hope* it will prevent disease. Even with vaccination, the possibility of the child getting that disease still remains. If a child may or may not get a disease in his lifetime, then vaccinating him to keep a disease away is based purely on *belief* or superstition.

There is a common thread of doubt that hangs over all childhood vaccines:

- Diseases declined before vaccines (so the credit for the lack of disease may be misplaced on vaccines).

- Children regularly get diseases for which they were vaccinated against (so one cannot claim that vaccines prevent disease).

- Vaccine damage statistics are manipulated and reporting of reactions and disease remains biased (so the understanding of the extent of vaccine damage and vaccine failure is elusive).

- All vaccines have documented harmful effects.

The vaccine philosophy perpetuates vaccination. It is rooted in strong cultural conditioning. Science's embrace of the germ theory lets everyone assume that germs attack at random and that there is little anyone can do about it. Taking full responsibility for the condition of the individual human body opens the door to better health. Through this awareness and acceptance, one can see that illness is simply a matter of how susceptible the body is made. One can make choices in his life that either prepares him for disease or builds for health.

Parents need time to make their choice regarding vaccines. During the decision-making process tremendous amounts of fear and anxiety play a role in which way they will lean. The impact of learning that vaccines may not be a good idea is profound enough, but actually making the choice *not* to vaccinate hurls them into a realm where seemingly "no man has gone before." This separates them from all the comforts of societal and cultural conditioning, so their convictions must be strong indeed in order to prevail. Parents will make a decision about childhood vaccines after much information-gathering, soul searching and an examination into how they choose to live their lives, based on their beliefs.

[This book focuses solely on the vaccines of childhood and how they relate to parents' decisions whether to give any or all to their children. Though there are many other vaccines for many other diseases (now and in the future), some experts would recommend that they also be scrutinized closely for their possible dangers.]

Part IV

The Parents' Decision

THE VACCINATION DECISION

- **Popular Questions**

- **Survey Results**
  - New Survey
  - Doubt
  - Regret
  - Intimidation
  - Family and Friends

- **It's Personal: Are you informed? Are you comfortable?**

- **Dear Doctor**

- **More Survey Quotes**

Popular Questions

The following actual questions are most often asked by parents struggling with the vaccine decision. The "answers" may help you with some of your own questions, enforce feelings you already have, or give you a firmer stand against opposite beliefs.

Can mass vaccinations eliminate childhood diseases?

Improved personal and public hygiene can account for a significant drop in deaths even before antibiotics or vaccines were introduced. In most cases, disease continued to decline at the same rate as before vaccines. Places *without* vaccination saw disease decline simultaneously with places that had the most vigorous vaccination programs. The introduction of vaccines may have been *coincidental* to the subsequent fall in disease rates. Many vaccines were introduced at a time when the disease would have been expected to decline anyway, so the question still remains as to whether vaccines could have a significant impact on the reduction of diseases.

Would epidemics return if vaccination stopped?

It has never been shown with any vaccine that during epidemics, those vaccinated were completely protected against that disease. Since both the vaccinated and unvaccinated get disease, then it cannot be assumed that vaccination plays a role in whether a disease might return. Halting vaccination would probably yield little change, and in some cases would lower disease rates.

If benefits outweigh the risks, then are vaccines better than nothing?

Other countries have abandoned certain vaccines after only a few cases of damage. The United States goes on and on, chalking up damage statistics and continuing to vaccinate in spite of evidence of vaccine injury. The incidence of the disease for which we vaccinate children has fallen so dramatically over the last century that it hardly justifies continuing in light of thousands of injuries from vaccines every year. In some cases, statistics show that indeed the *risks* outweigh the benefits. (See chapter on "The Benefits Outweigh the Risks?")

Is the risk of complication from a childhood disease greater than the risk of vaccination?

It is an error to state with any conviction or certainty that the benefits of vaccinating outweigh the risks, yet millions of children are vaccinated based on this *presumption*. The very diseases for which a person is vaccinated occur *regularly* in the same vaccinated population. Often 50% or more of the cases are in fully vaccinated individuals, so when vaccinating, there is the chance of getting the disease PLUS the chance of vaccine damage. Even when there is no obvious reaction from a vaccine, the fact cannot be overlooked that vaccines may be one cause of cancer and other chronic diseases involving immune failure. In actuality, the risk of several vaccines may indeed be greater than the risk of complication from a certain disease. (See chapter on "What Do Vaccines Do To The Body?")

Which vaccines are safest?

Some may seem to produce fewer side effects but no vaccine is guaranteed safe or effective. Doctors do not guarantee that there will be no side effects nor do they guarantee prevention of that disease. Manufacturers of vaccines extensively list possible adverse reactions and *never* make any guarantees. All vaccines have been linked to serious and/or deadly side effects. Many law suits have been settled and are pending regarding damage done in direct relationship to vaccines.

Do vaccines work?

In many cases, the disease rate is the same in those vaccinated as it is in those unvaccinated. So the idea that vaccines prevent disease is highly disputable. Besides, vaccines don't limit their activity to producing mild cases of disease, they all commonly produce a variety of symptoms of their own, sometimes producing slow viruses, sometimes death. If the vaccine just doesn't work, some feel at least they "tried." But what many do not realize is that if it doesn't work, they are not "even." They have *also* taken on substances that *must be dealt with* by the body. *Some* bodies cannot handle the intrusion and will suffer beyond any possible effects that may have occurred from the disease itself.

Are vaccines good preventive medicine?

It is highly questionable whether vaccines prevent disease because vaccinated individuals can contract the same disease they were vaccinated against. Vaccines carry risks of their own and it has been shown that disease declines among the unvaccinated at an equal pace as those vaccinated.

Isn't it unfair not to vaccinate because everyone should participate to make it work?

Each dose of each vaccine carries potential risks, so society does not benefit by one child taking unnecessary risks. Society would benefit if vaccines were always safe and effective but much evidence can show this is far from being the case. Since it is doubtful whether vaccines "work" in the first place, parents choosing not to vaccinate are making reasonable decisions that could actually be more beneficial to society in the long run.

Are unvaccinated children threatening the health of vaccinated children?

If a vaccinated child is assumed "protected" from that disease, then an unvaccinated child cannot possibly pose a threat.

What about the polio epidemic?

Many people have memories of the polio epidemic of the 1950's or have a family member who was affected, or may know someone whose relative died. This historical event alone can send an otherwise skeptical person into a doctor's office for the polio vaccine. The vaccine offered hope in the face of despair. In the people's impatience for a cure or something to "do" about this, almost anything was worth trying, even if that meant risking danger beyond what the disease already had to offer. The early controversy over the vaccine is kept out of modern-day questioning. In the 50's many people rejected the polio vaccine for fear it was causing polio. Statistics show a decline in polio *previous* to the introduction of widespread polio vaccination. It becomes clear that polio vaccination is continued as a result of incomplete information and is based on fears of yesterday. The controversies raging in the 50's are erased, and as a result the vaccine becomes unanimously accepted. (See chapter on "Polio")

I live on a farm and I am afraid of my child getting tetanus.

A person has a 180 times greater chance of dying from tuberculosis than from tetanus. Tetanus cannot be gotten from a "rusty nail" alone. The fatality rate for children is lower than in adults, but far, far below the 50-50 chance of dying that is often portrayed. Good wound hygiene could do more to prevent tetanus than the vaccine. Some people who get tetanus have been previously vaccinated and some previously vaccinated people die from tetanus. This disease probably causes more fear in parents than all the other vaccinated diseases so for this reason, vaccines can be "sold" to frightened and uninformed parents. (See chapter on "Tetanus")

Why not give a vaccine just to be sure? For "peace of mind?"

You cannot be sure *beforehand* that it would not also cause serious damage. Damage has been documented and much remains to be understood about exactly what vaccines do to the body. Some gain "peace of mind" by knowing they have not been responsible for crippling their child as the result of a vaccine.

Why not simply postpone the vaccines until the baby is older?

Many parents who first encounter doubts about vaccinating feel that this is a reasonable approach. While for the most part, vaccine reactions could be less severe in an older baby, one must still consider the overall impact on the human immune system. And after waiting a year (for example) before vaccinating, a person may feel that now the baby is also past a point when he would be the most vulnerable to complications from a disease. So the "reasons for vaccinating" start to become less and less significant as time goes on.

If my child did "OK" after one shot, then why should I worry?

A body is programmed to rid itself of foreign invasions. The healthy body will always react to a vaccine. The toxins in a vaccine are foreign to human beings and in the body's effort to rid itself of the poisons, shows symptoms like fever, swelling, etc. After the initial impact of the first vaccine, the body may have been weakened (See chapter on "Why Do Vaccines Appear to Work? — Tolerance") to such a degree that it is no longer able to muster the same acute response as it did initially to clear it of the invasion. Some children who have been vaccinated once without obvious damaging effects end up severely damaged or dead after either the second, third, fourth or fifth shot.

What if I start vaccines? Shouldn't I finish?

First, form your opinions objectively. If you decide vaccines are not a good idea, then you can assume if any are bad, then fewer are better. Remember, many children suffer permanent damage or death, not after the first vaccine, but after subsequent doses.

What if I start vaccines and then change my mind, is there anything I can do to reverse possible damage?

The first thing you should do after changing your mind is be thankful that at least you cannot see any apparent damage and if there is damage, be thankful you still have your child. Then, talk about it. Let your friends and family know what happened or what could have happened to your child and why. Give them information. Tell them that you are concerned for all children's safety. Also, maintaining a good diet and low stress environment can, not only prevent disease, but also reverse damage to the immune system.

How would I feel if my child gets something I did not vaccinate for?

There are many dangerous diseases for which there is no vaccine. The very existence of a vaccine makes one have more fear of *that* disease. Objectively speaking, one should not have different emotions toward vaccinated diseases than toward non-vaccinated diseases. But the idea that a vaccine may have prevented a disease has been planted in most people's minds, thereby creating a notion that one would feel guilty if their child contracted a disease for which there is a vaccine. Another question to ask would be: "What if my child were damaged by a vaccine? How would I feel?" If your child catches a disease normally vaccinated against, you may wonder if your child had a particular susceptibility to that disease. If that were true, then could a dose of the same virus also have caused the child problems?

The diseases for which there is a vaccine that you are most likely to encounter are pertussis and measles. When family and friends know you have not vaccinated your child, you would probably suffer scorn if your child contracted one of these diseases. This is part of the reason you must become strengthened in your decisions. Remind them and yourself that, vaccinated children get pertussis and measles too. *Vaccinated kids get it too!*

Can I be sure my child will remain healthy if he is not vaccinated?

With the growing concern over the dangers of vaccines, many people are returning to the "old fashioned" ways of preventing illness in their family: healthy diet, clean living and a low stress environment. Since the same diseases occur in both the vaccinated and unvaccinated, it is questionable whether vaccines are responsible for maintaining health in the first place.

Do I have to be more careful about health because my children are not vaccinated?

Somehow parents think they are on thin ice if they choose not to vaccinate. They feel that they are more vulnerable to disease without the interference of man's technologies. One may choose to be more careful and health conscious because he doesn't vaccinate, and that may make him *feel* better or make others feel better about him. But it is always wise to be careful about hygiene, diet, etc. whether vaccinating or not. If someone has come to believe that vaccines are ineffective and/or cause harm, then going without cannot *make* one more vulnerable to anything.

The fact that a person feels "special" or more vulnerable without vaccines shows there is still a shadow of doubt about their decision not to vaccinate. Still in their mind is the possibility that vaccines could actually provide a positive benefit. In every other aspect of life, simple decisions are made: "Does this product work for me? Does it do what it says it will? If it doesn't, I will stop buying it. If I find it causes harm (allergy, accident, etc.) I will reject it." We have no hesitation about these decisions. They are made objectively based on what is known about results. With vaccines, it is the deep desire of *wanting* them to work that causes anxiety. If you believe that the condition of the body is of key importance when determining the likelihood of whether one will become ill or not, then you will want to maintain health by building the immune system and having it ready for *any* intrusion that may occur. Singling out certain diseases and manipulating the immune system in order that it *might* prevent those diseases is pure vaccine philosophy and not an understanding of health in general.

If vaccines are so dangerous, why don't I know anyone who has ever had a reaction to a vaccine?

We also do not "see" many of the *diseases* vaccinated against, but still feel we must vaccinate. Just because damage is inapparent does not mean that it does not exist. Damage may be so subtle that even a close observer may miss it. Many parents are not informed about what a reaction would look like and many times when something is suspected, their doctor will deny any link to the vaccine. We see many diseases today that are related to chronic immune failure. We see children with chronic allergies (an immune dysfunction), we see recurrent ear infections, etc. With generations of people being subjected to the weakening of the immune system through vaccination, there is much speculation as to their full ramifications. Vaccines have proven to be dangerous and deadly in countless cases and how pervasive is the damage may never be known. By denying or minimizing the negative effects of vaccines, it belittles the countless children and their families who suffered and those who will surely suffer as vaccine practices continue. It also lessens the chance of ever finding the truth about vaccines or finding the true cause of many other diseases and conditions so familiar to the late 20th century. One organization, Dissatisfied Parents Together (see "Other Resources and Further Reading") makes it their job to offer medical, legal and moral support to those whose children have been damaged or killed by a vaccine. They have their hands full.

I am afraid to *not* vaccinate

It may seem better to just "grit your teeth" and hope that your child gets through it (vaccinating). The *brave* thing to do is what you see is right for your child, regardless of how your mother-in-law or your friends feel. Weighing whether or not to give vaccines goes beyond the fear of any given disease. Much of the fear may stem from the fact that when not vaccinating, it goes against the status quo and there is the feeling of having to defend your actions. You must try to separate your fear of disease from the fear of "being different." What are people going to think of you for being different? How do you reconcile that? Are you afraid of your own perceived future guilt if *your* child got sick? What are your *real* fears? Having opinions contrary to accepted societal philosophy automatically thrusts you into "unmapped territory" where you are usually left to find your way alone. Only you are the one ultimately responsible for your child. You have to live with any consequences that may result from your decisions.

Survey Results

During the last several years, parents were asked to respond to a survey. The parents' responses proved to be valuable in defining this book's direction and purpose in order to properly serve parents in particular, and anyone doubting vaccines.

The results are a sampling of parents most concerned about the vaccine issue. Some of the parents have a child who severely reacted to vaccines or who was damaged. But all of these parents wanted to share, hoping to help others in their decision-making.

Survey Results:

- *About half* of the parents never vaccinated their child.

- Of those who vaccinated *almost all* parents had doubts before, *all* had doubts after vaccinating and *all* regretted having ever vaccinated their child.

- *All* felt they were not given enough information by medical professionals.

- *Almost all* felt pressure and were victims of fear tactics in doctors' offices or clinics.

- *About half* felt intimidated when sharing their feelings on vaccines with family and friends.

- *All* needed and wanted more information to help them get closer to feeling comfortable with their decisions about vaccines (hence the fifth edition of *What About Immunizations?*).

Most parents reading this book can relate to all or most of these results. Actual quotes from the survey are interspersed throughout this chapter.

New Survey

If you would like to participate in a survey that may be used in future editions of *What About Immunizations?* please use another sheet of paper and answer the following questions. Be as brief or as thorough as you like. Your answers will be anonymous. Return to: Cynthia Cournoyer, 955 SW Central Ave., Grants Pass, OR 97526.

1. If you never vaccinated a child, what source of information did you find most helpful?

2. If you started the vaccines why did you go ahead?

3. If you started and then stopped, what most significantly attributed to your decision?

4. When did you first have doubts about vaccines?

5. If your child experienced a reaction to the vaccines, describe (confirmed by physicians or by your own beliefs).

6. What conversations have you had with medical personnel?

7. Do you feel you were properly informed by authorities on vaccines?

8. What other information about vaccines would you find helpful?

9. Have vaccines and school entry been a problem?

10. Do you share your feelings on the subject of vaccines with family and friends?

Doubt

Everybody: Vaccines are good!
Parent: I doubt it. I choose to *not* vaccinate my children.
Everybody: It's wrong to not vaccinate!
Parent: I doubt my decision to not vaccinate.
Friend: Vaccines could harm your child.
Parent: OK, I won't vaccinate my child.
Everybody: Your child could get sick!
Parent: I'm afraid of disease, OK, I will vaccinate.
Friend: You need more information...

And so it goes...

Parents have serious doubts and legitimate concerns about vaccines, but when they choose the unvaccinated route, they doubt their decision. It goes around and around, their emotions and convictions fluctuating with the tide of who has the most influence upon them. Almost universally, those who ultimately chose not to vaccinate had some intuitive inkling that vaccinating is something they should not do. This is called their "original doubt."

The confusion enters when this original doubt is neither confirmed or properly addressed. What usually happens is that the parents begin to doubt their doubt.

There are two kinds of doubt: doubting that the wrong thing is right and doubting that the right thing is wrong. So it's no wonder that a parent can first have doubts that the vaccines are good and then go on to doubt their decision not to vaccinate! The desire to do what's best for their children causes parents enormous anxiety when contemplating the vaccine decision.

Society and a huge medical network pull parents in one direction and their doubt and common sense are pulling in another.

> "Everyone said one thing: vaccinate! But our instincts voiced doubts about it."

> "My first doubt surfaced when I imagined bringing my healthy baby into the doctor's office only to take her home crying with a fever. We were told how we could give certain doses of children's aspirin substitute to relieve pain and fever after the vaccines. I wanted to believe that doctors were in the business of keeping people healthy. It seemed so backwards. It was enough doubt to make us question the entire procedure. We left the doctor's office that day without the vaccines, feeling good our child was not crying or in pain, but uneasy about a decision that felt right at the time."

> "Injecting toxins into a healthy baby didn't make sense to me. How could it make my child healthier?"

117

"My own doubts always surface when this sensitive subject comes up. My goal is to become so informed that I'm not in question at all."

Regret

"I still regret going along with the established program. I continue to feel guilty [the child had a bad reaction] and am ashamed that I didn't go with my intuition which I always had done before and really do now! I wish I had done my parental homework! Aw, but such is hindsight!"

"We asked other parents and the majority of them did give shots and questioned the value of them afterwards."

"I am one of those parents who hadn't done my homework on immunizations before making my decision. There was also pressure to immunize our son from doctors and family. I just went along even though on a gut level, felt I shouldn't have."

"My instincts told me not to do it all along and afterwards I regretted it."

Parents come to regret their decision to vaccinate their child either after a severe reaction or after doing their "homework" and searching out some of the harder-to-find vaccine information. Almost all from the survey had previous doubts about vaccines when they felt it went against their common sense. Then, by their own account, this doubt was confirmed afterwards by guilt for having vaccinated.

It's amazing that some couples who go out of their way to become informed on such issues as childbirth and parenting, remain unaware of vaccine danger. It is by chance, by talking to a friend or by reading a magazine, not available on most newsstands, that they begin to dig deeply for seemingly hidden information.

"I would like to see information on vaccines more readily available in libraries and the health clinics should make information on the other side available. Too many people just are not aware of the research and information on the cons of immunization which is available. All they see are the pros and propaganda. It's really all quite sad and dangerous."

Intimidation

Parents trying to do the best for their children and who have legitimate concerns and gut level instincts telling them of vaccine dangers, are very often treated as ignorant or just another "hysterical" parent. With so many unanswered questions about vaccines and the immune system in general, even in the established medical literature, it is a shame that the vaccine philosophy is consistently forced on unsuspecting parents.

"Overall, I find medical professionals very unhelpful and narrow-minded about vaccines."

"I assumed they must work because I'd never heard anything bad about them."

"My husband questioned our pediatrician pretty extensively on immunizations. The doctor was visibly taken aback by the questions. Just like the government pamphlets, he offered no more information than that, which didn't satisfy our inquiries."

"It was just what you were supposed to do. I didn't know there could be a choice."

"I was led to believe immunizations were necessary."

"The pediatric nurse believes in the shots. She says they are a necessary evil."

"I didn't question anything and signed the warning sheet without reading it. I thought I was being a good mother."

"We realized there was a big fear thing placed on us."

"In the United States people are coerced into feeling afraid to even *consider* not immunizing children."

"I've had them [doctors] really scare me before I was more informed. They don't know about the truth, refuse to believe it, or think we are too dumb to understand the pros and cons of it."

"Medical people try to lay a really heavy guilt trip on you for not being faithful with the vaccines."

"My son's reactions to the DPT were all contraindications to further shots. Needless to say, I was ticked off that I had to find this out from a book [*DPT, A Shot in the Dark*] instead of my doctor being honest with me!"

"Our first pediatrician for our daughter was a woman. When I informed her we would not be needing them she began with the scare tactics and when she finally figured out that we weren't going to change our minds, and that we had done our homework, she blurted out, 'You're signing her death certificate if you don't get her immunized!' That was the last time we ever saw her."

Family and Friends

"This is a great way to become unpopular with the 'ignorance is bliss' types—no one likes a boat-rocker!"

"When I share my feelings on vaccines with family and friends, I'm cautious because people take offense and become defensive and uncomfortable."

"I am able to share my feelings about vaccines with very few of my family members because of the ingrained belief that I am not doing the right and beneficial thing. I have recently met many people that I am able to share my feelings with and are a great source of support for me. As for my friends of a long time, again I am not able to talk with many because there is a certain amount of fear and anger toward me for my decision."

"I share this information with *some* of my relatives and friends, the ones I think would be open-minded enough to understand and not think we're crazy!"

Parents who hold views other than the status quo are not only intimidated by medical professionals but very often by those who care about them the most. Family and friends must occasionally be sheltered from the truth about whether or not parents choose to vaccinate their children because of fear that it would cause unnecessary friction. The vaccine philosophy is so pervasive and so successful in rallying support that truly searching families can feel that they have been left out in the cold.

It's Personal

Are You Informed?

Most information readily available on vaccines is biased toward the vaccine philosophy. Ask yourself these questions and discover if you know the "other side" of the issue.

1. Am I aware of the dangers or lack of danger and number of cases each year for each disease?

2. Am I aware of the myths surrounding certain diseases?

3. Am I aware of the many possible dangers of vaccines?

4. Am I aware of the questionable record of vaccine safety and effectiveness?

5. Do I know my rights regarding vaccines and school entry?

6. Do I know options to traditional medicine?

7. Have I read other material available on the dangers of vaccines?

Are You Comfortable?

Making an informed decision is only half the battle. You must ultimately feel comfortable with your decision. When faced with opposition and your own doubts, it may make the difference in how easily you might be swayed. The following quiz was designed to help you see your own attitudes and opinions that may have a bearing on your decision.

Answer either "a" or "b" in each question. Choose the answer that most closely fits your feelings, lifestyle or choices you would likely make.

1. a. I believe diseases are wiped out by vaccines.

   b. I believe diseases have a natural rise and fall and many factors contribute to disease reduction.

2. a. I believe "germs" are the enemy, affecting people at random.

   b. I believe that "germs" can thrive only in an environment best suited for their growth. Each human being differs in his susceptibility.

3. a. I believe vaccines are preventive medicine.

   b. I believe good diet, good hygiene and a low stress environment are preventive medicine.

4. a. I believe my knowledge of hygiene and good diet is lacking and vaccines can compensate for poor diet and stressful living.

b.   I live a clean life in a healthy environment that includes a good diet, but vaccines further inhibit the body's own ability to fight infection anyway.

5. a.   I believe I am incapable of making a medical decision without the direct guidance of the traditional medical establishment. Health care should be left up to experts and no matter how much I read, they will have more right answers.

     b.   I believe that I am responsible for my child and that I must be capable of making informed medical decisions. No one knows my lifestyle and state of health of myself and children more intimately than I do and if further information is needed, I can rely on physicians for certain knowledge, but they should not and cannot make all decisions.

6. a.   I feel incapable of assessing the health of my child and must rely solely on doctors after the slightest deviation from perfect health.

     b.   I feel that my intuition goes a long way in telling me how severely ill my child may be. I monitor illness in my child carefully. I strive to become informed. I take responsibility for the illness and health of my child. I stay away from doctor's office visits as long as I feel comfortable doing so. A doctor's office visit is a fact-finding task to add to the knowledge I already have of my child. I use his information to further assess the condition and weigh the alternatives to various choices of treatment. I seek less invasive forms of treatment whenever possible.

7. a. I believe that I could not live with myself if I did not vaccinate and my child caught the disease. I would feel better about vaccine damage because I did "everything possible."

    b. Because illness occurs in both vaccinated and unvaccinated children, I believe I am willing to accept the consequences of a naturally occurring disease in my child and would prefer that to living with possible damage from the vaccine that I approved. I could not live with myself if my child was damaged by a vaccine that I authorized.

8. a. I believe I cannot live in this society without going along with well-accepted opinions. I would be uncomfortable by being different.

    b. I believe that I am capable of making my decisions regardless of societal pressure.

The more "b" answers that fit your philosophy and lifestyle, the closer you have become to feeling "comfortable" with a decision not to vaccinate.

Dear Doctor

Parents must realize that most doctors honestly *believe* that vaccines are truly safe and effective. Parents must respect the doctor's opinion while maintaining their own. Because of a doctor's automatic position of authority, parents easily slip into feeling inferior in their beliefs. Remember that doctors act on what they believe just as parents do. If doctors are sure vaccination is the *right* thing, they would want to do everything in their power to give the "best medical care." Similarly, if parents believe vaccines do more harm than good, then they will do what they must to protect their child.

This letter summarizes the feelings of many parents when making the decision not to vaccinate but still need to communicate with their child's doctor. It is provided for your use, in whole or in part. You may sign your name to it as you see fit.

Dear Doctor,

We, the parents of _____ need your compassion. We realize you are committed to the health of our child. But the child has been entrusted to us and we do not take this obligation lightly. We have done our "homework" and do not arrive at our decision irresponsibly. Much analysis, intellectual and spiritual, has gone into our search for direction on this issue. We have looked at vaccines from both sides and frankly, we are not happy with the lack of scientific validity and the many unanswered questions.

We cannot put our faith in medicine that works *some* of the time, *maybe*, and then also take the risk of vaccine damage. Because you see, if our child is damaged or killed by a vaccine, the benefit to *our* child is 0% and the risk is 100%. And since our child is dependent on us for nurturing and protection, it is incumbent upon us to protect our child from any *known* risks. There are known risks to vaccines and much evidence that discredits their overall safety and effectiveness. If, when you look at any vaccine study, you use the hypothesis: vaccines could be dangerous and have little or no effect, then vaccine failures will no longer be seen as flukes of nature, but as clues to what a disastrous form of "preventive medicine" they are.

The type of disease and the possible severity of a disease can't weigh as heavy because there are *many* diseases, just as horrible, for which there is no vaccine. So scaring us with the possible effects of a *certain* disease borders on unfair manipulation of our emotions.

Please consider that the built-in intelligence of the human immune system and other natural forms of preventive medicine might be the proper prescription for our family. You *know* you are taking a chance of vaccine damage with each and every dose you give. How can the chance of hurting *our* child "save" others? If you can see, even the slightest possibility that the "vaccine philosophy" has leaks in its arguments, then you will understand that we are filling in the gaps the best possible way we know how. Thank you for taking the time to hear our deepest and most sincere thoughts on the matter.

Sincerely,

Parents

More Survey Quotes

"We stopped vaccinating our son because our information was consistently telling us that we were doing a disservice to him."

"The more we looked into it, the more we found reasons not to go ahead with any vaccines ever!"

"I now have a fourth child who has never had any vaccination of any kind and will never, never receive one!"

COMPULSORY VACCINATION

- **School Entry**

- **Legal Help**

- **Religious Freedom**

- **Travel**

- **Perspective**

School Entry

Many parents find the question of school entry a heavy road-block in their search for answers. The public is almost never properly informed of vaccine exemptions. Basically, parents must remember there are many options available to them. Most importantly, the decision rests on the parents and they do not have to vaccinate their child in order to attend public school.

Your local school district may tell you the basic immunization laws, however, they tend to give simple statements like, "no shots, no school." You will need to read the law for yourself to determine *which* vaccines are actually required for school entry and which exemptions are allowed. For example, some states specifically disallow Naturopaths and Chiropractors from giving medical exemptions. Some make no mention of other physicians. Some require certain vaccines and not others. Some states require bonafide memberships in a certain religion before allowing religious exemptions and some will allow you to make religious statements without membership. Some have "conscientious objections," or "against personal beliefs" as exemptions.

States That Do Not Require *Petussis* Vaccination For School Entry (as of July 1989):

Arizona	Idaho	Kentucky
Missouri	Montana	New York
Oregon	Pennsylvania	Rhode Island
Texas	Washington	

States That Allow "Personal Conviction" Or "Philosophical Objection":

Arizona	California	Colorado
Delaware	Idaho	Indiana
Louisiana	Maine	Michigan
Minnesota	Missouri	Montana
Nebraska	North Dakota	Ohio
Oklahoma	Pennsylvania	Rhode Island
Utah	Vermont	Washington
Wisconsin		

In many of these states, a parent must object to all vaccines, not just a particular vaccine in order to use the "philosophical objection" or "personal conviction."

All Other States:

Most states (except Mississippi and West Virginia) will exempt a child from the vaccine requirement if the parents object on the grounds of *religious conviction.* Some states require the parent demonstrate belonging to a church whose religious beliefs specifically oppose vaccination. [283]

As state laws are always subject to revision, it is always wise to locate the precise law in your own state. Find the *Revised Statutes* in your library. Look in the index under either "Vaccines," "Immunizations," "Education," or "Schools." Also look in the back of the Index for updated revisions. Once in the correct volume, look for revisions in the back there also. The books are usually published only every several years. As the lawmakers revise or add laws, they are printed periodically and inserted in the back of these volumes.

Many states with religious and/or medical exemptions to "required" vaccines can legally exclude an unvaccinated student if there is an "outbreak" or an epidemic of a certain disease. This procedure has no sound basis and can be imposed quite arbitrarily. An "outbreak" can be defined after as few as eight cases of measles for example. The irony of this practice of exclusion is that *vaccinated* children are regularly victims of measles (for example) and if assuming that vaccines "work" then an unvaccinated child can be of no threat to others who are vaccinated. Also, the vaccinated child is *still* susceptible to the disease, the same as the unvaccinated child. It appears that the "outbreak" is simply the excuse to put more pressure on parents. Illogical assumptions and subjective enforcement of health laws are not uncommon.

If your child is excluded due to an "epidemic" ask for a private teacher. In a country where public education is every child's right, the school district should legally and gladly pay for this additional expense. There have been cases where a parent has contemplated suing the school district for interfering with the child's right to a free education.

Media exposure of the vaccine laws almost always neglects to mention any exemptions. The public is led to believe it is "against the law" to not vaccinate children before going to school. This leaves impressions of arrest and jail terms, and in fact some families have had to hire lawyers to protect their rights.

Currently, with more public awareness of the dangers and the visible recall of batches of DPT vaccines a few years ago, more and more parents are beginning to question the childhood vaccines and look for ways around the "compulsory" school entry laws.

Legal Help

Attorney Thomas G. Finn has litigated cases dealing with compulsory vaccination (see "Other Resources" for his book). He suggests that if an attorney is needed that he demand from the school board, the hospital and/or the physician administering the vaccine, a guarantee that the vaccine will not cause disease, death or injurious side effects, and that the vaccine will prevent the particular disease for which it is given to prevent. The guarantee should be worded in such a way that the person signing it is liable not only as a representative of the school district, etc. but also individually liable for any damages should they occur. To his knowledge, no one ever signed such a guarantee and in each case the child was allowed to return to school without the vaccines.

Compulsory immunization laws raise constitutional issues such as the violation of the First, Ninth, and Fourteenth Amendments as well as violation of civil tort law. [284]

Private schools can refuse admission to any child for any reason they choose. But refusal to admit a child on the basis of vaccine objections can create a legal liability for a private school in a state where religious or philosophical exemptions exist.

If a parent makes the choice to avoid vaccines, several court cases have provided precedents for a parent's right to make an informed decision about vaccines.

Religious Freedom

The United States Constitution does not define religion other than to allow "the free exercise thereof" and "Congress shall make no law respecting an establishment of religion..." States are prohibited from enacting laws that override federal laws. But when states respect one religion over another by defining religion by which is acceptable for required exemption to vaccination, they go against federal law.

Our *beliefs* are our religion. So we are guaranteed the freedom to exercise our beliefs. Recent legal precedents have established that religious belief may be personal and parents need not be associated with a religious institution opposed to vaccination. [285]

Travel

You may travel wherever you wish in the world without vaccines. The World Health Organization (WHO) in Geneva grants American visitors the right to refuse vaccines when traveling internationally. Thousands travel world-wide each year without vaccines. You can request a copy of "Foreign Rules and Regulations, Part 71, Title 42" on immunization when you receive your passport. Remember the basic rule that no one will vaccinate you against your will. [286]

When traveling, you can gain exemption from vaccines by referring to Clause 83 of the "International Sanitary Code," issued by the World Health Organization and adopted by all its members. It states that only when coming *from* an infected area are vaccinations necessary but the traveler has the option of being quarantined for up to 14 days from the time he left the infected area if the health department deems it necessary. If there has been an epidemic in an area that you're coming from, you could be put under surveillance. This means that together with the local health officer, you must keep a close watch for any suspicious signs or symptoms and report periodically for up to 14 days from the time of your departure from the infected area. If you notice any outbreak or symptom you must immediately turn yourself in and submit to quarantine or isolation. In actual practice this possibility is *very remote*. But if it should occur, *the vaccinated person may be required to submit to the same surveillance as the unvaccinated person!* [287]

Curiously enough, in 1975, while traveling in a foreign country, one man's experience may uncover yet another option. When it came time for the "required" vaccines, he simply explained it was against his religion. The official in charge made it very clear that he had no concern over whether the man got vaccinated but that he should *pay* for the vaccine anyway. The man paid his $2.00 and was on his way, unvaccinated. Ironically, third-world nations may be more interested in U.S. dollars than enforcing Western health "laws."

Perspective

As time goes on and more people become informed, the more absurd it will be that strict vaccination laws are allowed to exist (as in Mississippi and West Virginia, for example). The more we exercise our rights the more likely it is we will be able to keep them, and choices will be clear and tolerated. A country that prides itself on liberty should not rob freedom on a very basic and personal level: the freedom to shield our bodies from harmful toxins.

Parents who choose to keep their children unvaccinated are subject to harassment; they are accused of ignorance, fanaticism, and gross neglect, when in fact they are trying to follow their conscience and deep convictions concerning their child's health.

The government is asking us to take risks without choice. If compulsory vaccination laws are going to be enforced, then the public is surely entitled to convincing proof beyond reasonable doubt that vaccination is not only safe, but does what it was designed and advertised to do, and that absolutely no damaging effects could possibly result.

Today there is clearly no emergency reason why vaccination should be enforced. But there is clear evidence of vaccine dangers.

OTHER RESOURCES AND FURTHER READING

Helpful Organizations:

Dissatisfied Parents Together (DPT)
128 Branch Rd., Vienna, VA 22180
(703) 938-DPT3

> This organization was instrumental in gaining support for the National Childhood Vaccine Injury Act. Along with many lay people and professionals in the legal and medical fields, they continue to offer medical, legal and moral support for any family injured or concerned about childhood vaccines.

Vaccination Alternatives
Sharon Kimmelman
PO Box 346, New York, NY 10023
(212) 870-5117

> Vaccine information pack is available through Vaccination Alternatives. Includes an extensive list of other sources (books, articles, audiotapes, etc.) on vaccines and health.

What About Immunizations?

National Center for Homeopathy
1500 Massachusetts Ave., NW, Suite 42, Washington, D.C. 20005
(202) 223-6182

> A national directory of homeopathic practitioners is available through this information resource center for homeopathic medicine.

Available Through Your Bookstore:

Immunization: The Reality Behind the Myth
by Walene James, with a forward by Robert S. Mendelsohn
Bergin & Garvey, Publishers, Inc., 1988

The Immunization Decision: A Guide for Parents
by Randall Neustaedter
North Atlantic Books, 1990

How to Raise a Healthy Child... In Spite of Your Doctor
by Robert S. Mendelsohn
Now available in pocketbook

Other Publications:

DPT: A Shot in the Dark
by Harris L. Coulter and Barbara Loe Fisher: $9.00
Dissatisfied Parents Together (DPT)
128 Branch Rd., Vienna, VA 22180

Whooping Cough, the DPT Vaccine and Reducing Vaccine Reactions
Parent's Information Packet: $5.00
National Vaccine Information Center
128 Branch Rd., Vienna, VA 22180

134

Immunity, Why Not Keep It?
by Lisa Lovett, D.C.: $12.00
86 Kooyong Rd., Armdale, Victoria, 3143 Australia

The Case Against Immunizations
by Richard Moskowitz, M.D.: $2.25
National Center for Homeopathy
1500 Massachusetts Ave., NW, Washington, DC 20005

Immunization: An Informed Choice
by Daniel A. Lander: $2.20
Daniel A. Lander, Family Chiropractor
Rt. 1, Box 109, Glen Cove, ME 04846

Dangers of Compulsory Immunizations, How to Avoid Them Legally
by Attorney Tom Finn: $5.95
Family Fitness Press
PO Box 1658, New Port Richey, FL 33552

Immunization Booklet
$7.00:
Mothering Publications
PO Box 8410, Santa Fe, NM 87504

Three booklet set:
The Dangers of Immunization
Vaccinations and Immune Malfunction
How to Legally Avoid Unwanted Immunizations of All Kinds
$9.00 for all three:
Humanitarian Publishing Co.
RD 3, Clymer Rd., Quakertown, PA 18951

What About Immunizations?

Immunization Kit
$5.00:
The National Health Federation
PO Box 688, Monrovia, CA 91016

AIDS and Vaccination: The London Times Reports
by Gene Franks: $4.00
Pure Water Products
Box 2783, Denton, TX 76201

AIDS: The Alarming Reality
by William T. O'Connor, M.D.: $5.00
The H.I.V.E. Foundation
PO Box 808, Vacaville, CA 95696

AIDS: The End of Civilization
by William Campbell Douglass, M.D.: $9.95
Valet Publishers
PO Box 1568, Clayton, GA 30525

Natural Treatment for Childhood Diseases
by Stan Malstrom, N.D., M.T.: $3.95
Economy Herbs
Box 587, Melbourne, AR 72556

The "Natural Hygienic" principles of Superior Nutrition. *Food Combining Simplified* and *Maximizing Your Nutrition*
Two book set, $8.00:
D. Nelson
P.O. Box 2302, Santa Cruz, CA 95063

Periodicals...

The People's Doctor Newsletter
by Robert S. Mendelsohn
The Risks of Immunizations and How to Avoid Them: A collection of 13 newsletters dealing with vaccines.
100 page booklet with a complete index.
$15.00:
The Doctor's People
1578 Sherman, Ave., Suite 318, Evanston, IL 60201

East/West Journal
"How We Beat the School System — One Family's Lengthy Struggle to Avoid Compulsory Immunizations at School," by Robert Allanson, November 1984.
Reprint:
"Who Calls the Shots?: The Vaccination Debate," November 1988.
$3.00 each:
East/West Journal
Back Issues Dept. 144B
17 Station St., PO Box 1200, Brookline, MA 02147

"Children at Risk: The DPT Dilemma"
Tabloid reprint of a series of articles
by Jennifer Hyman (Excellent): $3.00:
Rochester Democrat and Chronicle
55 Exchange Blvd., Rochester, NY 14614-2001

The Vaccine Machine
Special Report: FREE
Gannett News Service
Box 7858, Washington, D.C. 20044

What About Immunizations?

DPT
Special Tabloid: FREE
The Fresno Bee
1626 E Street, Fresno, CA 93786

Transcripts...

DPT: Vaccine Roulette and DPT: One Year Later
Transcripts of broadcasts on April 19, 1982, and May 11, 12, 13, &
16, 1983.
WRC-TV, Washington D.C.
$5.00 for both:
National Broadcasting Company, Inc. (NBC)
4001 Nebraska Ave., NW, Washington, D.C. 20016

20/20 on the DPT Shot
Transcript of the broadcast in April 1985
$3.00:
ABC News
Transcript #505
Box 2020 Ansonia Station, New York, NY 10023

138

Videos...

The Strecker Memorandum
by Robert B. Strecker, M.D.
Well documented 90 minute video of the characteristics of the AIDS virus and how it was likely produced.
$29.95:
The Strecker Group
1216 Wilshire Blvd., Los Angeles, CA 90017
(213) 977-1210

AIDS: The World is Dying for the Truth
by William T. O'Connor, M.D. and others
Discusses the political and public health response to the AIDS epidemic.
$29.95:
Rod Blanchard & Associates
1042 E. Fort Union Blvd., Suite 367, Salt Lake City, UT 84047

FOOTNOTES

1. E.D. Shapiro and A.T. Berg, "Protective Efficacy of Haemophilus Influenza Type B Polysaccharide Vaccine." *Pediatrics, supplement to, part 2, Current Status of Haemophilus Influenzae type b Vaccines*, vol. 85, No. 4. (American Academy of Pediatrics, April 1990).

2. Drs. E. Cheraskin and W.M. Ringsdorf, Jr. from their book *Psychodietetics*, as quoted by Hannah Allen, *Don't Get Stuck!*

3. Walene James, *Immunization: The Reality Behind the Myth*, with a forward by Robert S. Mendelsohn, M.D. (Massachusetts: Bergin & Garvey Publishers, Inc., 1988).

4. Ibid.

5. Ibid.

6. Ibid.

7. Hannah Allen, *Don't Get Stuck.* (Natural Hygiene Press, PO Box 1083, Oldsmar, FL 33557, 1985).

8. Ibid.

9. Ibid.

10. Ibid.

11. Ibid.

12. Harold E. Buttram, M.D. and John Chriss Hoffman, *Vaccinations and Immune Malfunction.* (Humanitarian Publishing Co., RD Burleson Rd., Austin, TX 78744, 1982).

13. *The Burbank Leader*, April 15, 1987, Burbank, California.

14. Hannah Allen, *Don't Get Stuck!*

15. *Immunizations, Special Edition.* (Mothering Publications, PO Box 1690, Santa Fe, NM 87504, 1984).

16. Hannah Allen, *Don't Get Stuck.*

17. Walene James, *Immunization: The Reality Behind the Myth.*

18. *Immunizations, Special Edition.* (Mothering Publications).

19. Hannah Allen, *Don't Get Stuck.*

20. Walene James, *Immunization: The Reality Behind the Myth.*

21. Ibid.

22. *Immunizations, Special Edition.* (Mothering Publications).

23. Hannah Allen, *Don't Get Stuck.*

24. Walene James, *Immunization: The Reality Behind the Myth.*

25. Ibid.

26. Ibid.

27. Randall Neustaedter, *The Immunization Decision: A Guide for Parents.* (The Family Health Series, North Atlantic Books, 2800 Woolsey Street, Berkeley, CA 94705, 1990).

28. Walene James, *Immunization: The Reality Behind the Myth.*

29. Ibid.

30. Ibid.

31. Ibid.

32. Harris L. Coulter and Barbara Loe Fisher, *DPT, A Shot in the Dark.* (Warner Books, PO Box 690, New York, NY 10019, 1985).

33. Walene James, *Immunization: The Reality Behind the Myth.*

34. E. McBean, Ph,D., N.D., *Vaccinations Do Not Protect.* (The Health Library, 6600-D, Burleson Rd., Austin, TX 78744, 1980).

35. Harold E. Buttram, M.D., *Vaccinations and Immune Malfunction.*

36. Lawrence K. Altman, "New Whooping Cough Vaccines: Promise Dims." *New York Times,* May 10, 1988, C3.

37. Walene James, *Immunization: The Reality Behind the Myth.*

38. Richard Moskowitz, M.D., *The Case Against Immunizations.* (National Center for Homeopathy, 1500 Massachusetts Ave., NW, Washington, D.C. 20005).

39. George Vithoulkas, *The Science of Homeopathy.* (Grove Press Inc., 196 W. Houston St., New York, NY 10014, 1980).

40. Ibid.

41. Ibid.

42. *The Dangers of Immunization.* (Humanitarian Publishing Co., RD 3, Clymer Rd., Quakertown, PA 18951, 1983).

43. Hannah Allen, *Don't Get Stuck.*

44. Ibid.

45. E. McBean, *Vaccinations Do Not Protect.*

46. Richard Moskowitz, M.D., *The Case Against Immunizations.*

47. Hannah Allen, *Don't Get Stuck.*

48. Ibid.

49. *Immunizations, Special Edition.* (Mothering Publications).

50. Ibid.

51. Elben, *Vaccination Condemned*. (Better Life Research, PO Box 42002, Los Angeles, CA 90042, 1981).

52. *Physician's Desk Reference* (PDR), 1990, p. 1151, 2363.

53. *Immunization Kit*. (The National Health Federation, PO Box 688, Monrovia, CA 91016).

54. *Immunizations, Special Edition*. (Mothering Publications).

55. *Physician's Desk Reference* (PDR), 1990, p. 1401, 1402.

56. Gene Franks, *AIDS and Vaccinations, The London Times Reports*. (Pure Water Products, Box 2783, Denton, TX 76201, 1988).

57. Elben, *Vaccination Condemned*.

58. S. Lavi, "Administration of Measles, Mumps, and Rubella Virus Vaccine (Live) to Egg-Allergic Children." *Journal of the American Medical Association*. 1990; 263:269.

59. Ibid.

60. Walene James, *Immunization: The Reality Behind the Myth*.

61. Richard Moskowitz. M.D., *The Case Against Immunizations*.

62. Walene James, *Immunization: The Reality Behind the Myth*.

63. *The Dangers of Immunization*.

64. *Immunizations, Special Edition*. (Mothering Publications).

65. *The Dangers of Immunization*.

66. Richard Moskowitz, M.D., *The Case Against Immunizations*.

67. Robert S. Mendelsohn, M.D., "Recent Immunization Research." *People's Doctor Newsletter*, Vol. 6, No. 12, PO Box 982, Evanston, IL 60204.

68. *The Dangers of Immunization*.

69. Ibid.

70. Hannah Allen, *Don't Get Stuck*.

71. *The Dangers of Immunization*.

72. Randall Neustaedter, *The Immunization Decision: A Guide for Parents*.

73. *The Dangers of Immunizations*.

74. Richard Moskowitz, M.D., *The Case Against Immunizations*.

75. Robert S. Mendelsohn, M.D., "Recent Immunization Research."

76. Richard Moskowitz, M.D., *The Case Against Immunizations*.

77. Randall Neustaedter, *The Immunization Decision: A Guide for Parents*.

78. *Whooping Cough, the DPT Vaccine and Reducing Vaccine Reactions*. (National Vaccine Information Center, 128 Branch Road, Vienna, VA 22180).

79. Harris L. Coulter, *DPT, A Shot in the Dark*.

80. Randy Neustaedter, with revisions and additions by Steve Cummings, Greg Manteuffel, M.D., and Dennis Chernin, M.D., *Immunizations: Are They Necessary?* (The Hering Family Health Clinic, 2340 Ward St., Suite 107, Berkeley, CA 94705, 1977, second edition 1981).

81. Harris L. Coulter, *DPT: A Shot in the Dark.*

82. Jennifer Hyman, "Children at Risk: the DPT Dilemma." *The Democrat & Chronicle*, 55 Exchange Blvd., Rochester, NY 14614-2001, Special Report, April 1987.

83. Harris L. Coulter, *DPT: A Shot in the Dark.*

84. Jennifer Hyman, "Children at Risk: the DPT Dilemma."

85. Ibid.

86. Ibid.

87. Ibid.

88. Ibid.

89. *Immunizations, Special Edition.* (Mothering Publications).

90. Jennifer Hyman, "Children at Risk: the DPT Dilemma."

91. *Whooping Cough, the DPT Vaccine and Reducing Vaccine Reactions.*

92. *Lancet*, April 30, 1988:955.

93. Jennifer Hyman, "Children at Risk: the DPT Dilemma."

94. *Whooping Cough, the DPT Vaccine and Reducing Vaccine Reactions.*

95. Ibid.

96. Ibid.

97. Ibid.

98. Ibid.

99. Ibid.

100. Robert S. Mendelsohn, M.D., "The Truth About Immunizations." *The People's Doctor Newsletter*, Vol. 2, No. 4.

101. Harris L. Coulter, *DPT: A Shot in the Dark.*

102. Jennifer Hyman, "Children at Risk: the DPT Dilemma."

103. M.R. Griffin, et al., "Risk of SIDS After Immunization with DPT Vaccine." *New England Journal of Medicine*, Sept. 8, 1988, Vol. 319, No. 10, p. 618-622.

104. Randall Neustaedter, *The Immunization Decision: A Guide for Parents.*

105. Jennifer Hyman, "Children at Risk: the DPT Dilemma."

106. *DPT News*, Vol. 3, No. 2, Summer/Fall 1987. (DPT, 128 Branch Rd., Vienna, VA 22180).

107. Jennifer Hyman, "Children at Risk: the DPT Dilemma."

108. Ibid.

109. *Whooping Cough, the DPT Vaccine and Reducing Vaccine Reactions.*

110. Harris L. Coulter, *DPT: A Shot in the Dark.*

111. Jennifer Hyman, "Children at Risk: the DPT Dilemma."

112. Harris L. Coulter, *DPT: A Shot in the Dark.*

113. Jennifer Hyman, "Children at Risk: the DPT Dilemma."

114. *DPT News.*

115. Jennifer Hyman, "Children at Risk: the DPT Dilemma."

116. Robert S. Mendelsohn, M.D., "Recent Immunization Research."

117. Jennifer Hyman, "Children at Risk: the DPT Dilemma."

118. *Whooping Cough, the DPT Vaccine and Reducing Vaccine Reactions.*

119. Ibid.

120. *MMWR.* 1990; 39: 57-66.

121. Ibid.

122. *Whooping Cough, the DPT Vaccine and Reducing Vaccine Reactions.*

123. Harris L. Coulter, *DPT: A Shot in the Dark.*

124. Robert S. Mendelsohn, M.D., "Recent Immunization Research."

125. Jennifer Hyman, "Children at Risk: the DPT Dilemma."

126. Ibid.

127. Ibid.

128. G.R. Noble, R.H. Bernier, E.C. Esber, et al. "Acellular and Whole-Cell pertussis vaccines in Japan: Report of a visit by U.S. scientists." *Journal of the American Medical Association* 1987; 257:1351-1356, as cited by Randall Neustaedter, *The Immunization Decision: A Guide For Parents.*

129. Jennifer Hyman, "Children at Risk: the DPT Dilemma."

130. M. Blennow and M. Granstrom, "Adverse reactions and serologic response to a booster dose of acellular pertussis vaccine in children immunized with acellular or whole-cell vaccine as infants." *Pediatrics* 1989; 84:62-67, as cited by Randall Neustaedter, *The Immunization Decision: A Guide for Parents.*

131. Randall Neustaedter, *The Immunization Decision: A Guide For Parents.*

132. Robert S. Mendelsohn, M.D., "Immunization Update." *The People's Doctor Newsletter*, Vol. 10, No. 5.

133. Randy Neustaedter, *Immunizations: Are They Necessary?*

134. Elben, *Vaccination Condemned.*

135. *The Dangers of Immunizations.*

136. Elben, *Vaccination Condemned.*

137. Randy Neustaedter, *Immunizations: Are They Necessary?*

138. "Tetanus — United States, 1986." *MMWR*, 1987; 36:477-481, as cited by Randall Neustaedter, *The Immunization Decision: A Guide For Parents.*

139. Randy Neustaedter, *Immunizations: Are They Necessary?*

140. *Mosby's Medical and Nursing Dictionary* (1983), p. 1063.

141. Randall Neustaedter, *The Immunization Decision: A Guide For Parents.*

142. "Tetanus — United States, 1987 and 1988." *MMWR*, January 26, 1990; 39:37-41.

143. Ibid.

144. "Tetanus — United States, 1986." *MMWR* 1987; 36:477-481, as cited by Randall Neustaedter, *The Immunization Decision: A Guide For Parents.*

145. Randall Neustaedter, *The Immunization Decision: A Guide For Parents.*

146. "Cases of specified notifiable diseases, United States, weeks ending December 16, 1989 and December 17, 1988 (50th week)." *MMWR* 1989; 38:869.

147. "Tetanus — United States, 1987 and 1988." *MMWR*, January 26, 1990; 39:37-41.

148. Skudder and McCarroll, *Journal of the American Medical Association*, 1964, as cited by Randall Neustaedter, *The Immunization Decision: A Guide For Parents.*

149. *Physician's Desk Reference*, 1990.

150. Robert S. Mendelsohn, M.D., "More Anti-Vaccine Arguments." *The People's Doctor Newsletter*, Vol. 6, No. 12.

151. Idem. "Immunization Update." *The People's Doctor Newsletter*, Vol. 10, No. 5.

152. "Tetanus — United States, 1987 and 1988." *MMWR*, January 26, 1990; 39:37-41.

153. Robert S. Mendelsohn, M.D., "... Polio Vaccine." *The People's Doctor Newsletter*, Vol. 9, No. 2

154. "Rubella and congenital rubella syndrome — United States, 1985-1988." *MMWR* 1989; 38:173-178, as cited by Randall Neustaedter, *The Immunization Decision: A Guide For Parents.*

155. Randall Neustaedter, *The Immunization Decision: A Guide For Parents.*

156. *Physician's Desk Reference*, 1990, p. 1401.

157. Robert S. Mendelsohn, M.D., "Avoiding Immunizations and Their Dangers." *The People's Doctor Newsletter*, Vol. 7, No. 10.

158. Walene James, *Immunization: The Reality Behind the Myth.*

159. Robert S. Mendelsohn, M.D., "More Vaccine Arguments." *The People's Doctor Newsletter*, Vol. 8, No. 12.

160. *Immunization Kit.*

161. *Immunizations, Special Edition.* (Mothering Publications)

162. V.A. Fulginiti, "Controversies in current immunization policies and practices. Current Problems in Pediatrics 1976"; 6:6-16, as cited by Randall Neustaedter, *The Immunization Decision: A Guide For Parents.*

163. Randall Neustaedter, *The Immunization Decision: A Guide For Parents.*

164. Joseph A. Bellanti, M.D. and John B. Robbins, M.D., *Immunology III; Immunoprophylaxis: The Use of Vaccines.* Chapter 23. (W.B. Sauders Company, 1985).

165. Chester A. Wilk, D.C., *Chiropractic Speaks Out.*

166. Lisa Lovett, D.C., David M. Lovett, D.C., Cynthia Lovett-O'Meara, B.Sc (Nut), *Immunity, Why Not Keep It?* (Technical Publications Pty. Ltd., 15 - 17 Normanby Rd., Clayton, Victoria, 3168, Australia).

167. Robert S. Mendelsohn, M.D., "Immunization Update." *The People's Doctor Newsletter*, Vol. 4, No. 5.

168. "Rubella and congenital rubella syndrome — United States, 1985-1988." MMWR 1989; 38:173-178, as cited by Randall Neustaedter, *The Immunization Decision: A Guide For Parents.*

169. Randy Neustaedter, *Immunizations: Are They Necessary?*

170. *Lancet*, October 28, 1989, p. 1015.

171. Randy Neustaedter, *Immunizations: Are They Necessary?*

172. Idem. *The Immunization Decision: A Guide For Parents.*

173. Ibid.

174. Robert S. Mendelsohn, M.D., "Immunization Update." *The People's Doctor Newsletter*, Vol. 4, No. 5.

175. *Lancet*, October 28, 1989, p. 1015.

176. Ibid.

177. *Immunizations, Special Edition.* (Mothering Publications).

178. Lisa Lovett, D.C., *Immunity, Why Not Keep It?*

179. Randall Neustaedter, *The Immunization Decision: A Guide For Parents.*

180. Harold E. Buttram, M.D., *Vaccinations and Immune Malfunction.*

181. Randall Neustaedter, *The Immunization Decision: A Guide For Parents.*

182. Joseph A. Bellanti, M.D. and John B. Robbins, M.D., *Immunology III; Immunoprophylaxis: The Use of Vaccines.*

183. Robert S. Mendelsohn, M.D., The Truth About Immunizations. *The People's Doctor Newsletter*, Vol. 2, No. 4.

184. *Physician's Desk Reference (PDR) 1990.*

185. Elben, *Vaccinations Condemned.*

186. J.D. Cherry, R.D. Feigin, L.A. Lobes, P.G. Shackelford. "Atypical measles in children previously immunized with attenuated measles virus vaccines." *Pediatrics* 1972; 50:712, as cited by Randall Neustaedter, *The Immunization Decision: A Guide For Parents.*

187. J.W. St. Gene, B.L. George, B.M Bush. "Exaggerated natural measles following attenuated virus immunization." *Pediatrics* 1976; 57:148-150, as cited by Randall Neustaedter, *The Immunization Decision: A Guide For Parents.*

188. Hannah Allen, *Don't Get Stuck.*

189. L.E. Markowitz, S.R. Preblud, W.A. Orenstein, et al. "Patterns of transmission in measles outbreaks in the United States, 1985-1986." *New England Journal of Medicine* 1989; 320:75-81, as cited by Randall Neustaedter, *The Immunization Decision: A Guide For Parents.*

190. M.B. Edmonson, et al. "Mild measles and secondary vaccine failure during a sustained outbreak in a highly vaccinated population." *Journal of the American Medical Association*, May 9, 1990; 263:2467-2471.

191. "Measles." *MMWR* 1989; 38:329-330.

192. "Measles, Quebec." *MMWR* 1989; 38:329-330.

193. *MMWR.* February 1985, as cited by Lisa Lovett, D.C., *Immunity, Why Not Keep It?*

194. L.E. Markowitz, S.R. Preblud, W.A. Orenstein, et al. "Patterns of transmission in measles outbreaks in the United States, 1985-1986." *New England Journal of Medicine* 1989; 320:75-81, as cited by Randall Neustaedter, *The Immunization Decision: A Guide For Parents.*

195. M.B. Edmonson, et al. "Mild measles and secondary vaccine failure during a sustained outbreak in a highly vaccinated population." *Journal of the American Medical Association*, May 9, 1990; 263:2467-2471.

196. Randall Neustaedter, *The Immunization Decision: A Guide For Parents.*

197. "Answering Immunization Questions," *The Doctor's People*, Vol. 3, No. 2 (February 1990): p. 4-6.

198. *Immunization Kit.*

199. Randy Neustaedter, *Immunizations: Are They Necessary?*

200. Idem. *The Immunization Decision: A Guide For Parents.*

201. Idem. *Immunizations: Are They Necessary?*

202. *Immunization Kit.*

203. *The Dangers of Immunizations.*

204. *Immunization Kit.*

205. Randall Neustaedter, *The Immunization Decision: A Guide For Parents.*

206. *Immunizations, Special Edition.* (Mothering Publications).

207. *The Dangers of Immunizations.*

208. *Immunization Kit.*

209. Walene James, *Immunization: The Reality Behind the Myth.*

210. *The Dangers of Immunization.*

211. Walene James, *Immunization: The Reality Behind the Myth.*

212. Randy Neustaedter, *Immunizations: Are They Necessary?*

213. Lisa Lovett, D.C., *Immunity, Why Not Keep It?*

214. Randy Neustaedter, *Immunizations: Are They Necessary?*

215. Robert S. Mendelsohn, M.D., "Immunization Update." *The People's Doctor Newsletter*, Vol. 10, No. 5.

216. Walene James, *Immunization: The Reality Behind the Myth.*

217. Ibid.

218. *Physician's Desk Reference,* 1990, p. 1173.

219. E. McBean, *Vaccinations Do Not Protect.*

220. *Immunizations, Special Edition,* p. 24. (Mothering Publications).

221. Robert S. Mendelsohn, M.D., "... Polio Vaccine." *The People's Doctor Newsletter*, Vol. 9, No. 2.

222. Randy Neustaedter, *Immunizations: Are They Necessary?*

223. Ibid.

224. Daniel A. Lander, *Immunization: An Informed Choice.* (Family Chiropractor, Rt., 1, box 109, Glen Cove, ME 04846).

225. Randy Neustaedter, *Immunizations: Are They Necessary?*

226. Robert S. Mendelsohn, M.D., "… Polio Vaccine."

227. Randall Neustaedter, *The Immunization Decision: A Guide For Parents.*

228. Jennifer Hyman, "Children at Risk: the DPT Dilemma."

229. Randall Neustaedter, *The Immunization Decision: A Guide For Parents.*

230. *Immunization Kit.*

231. Randy Neustaedter, *Immunizations: Are They Necessary?*

232. Idem. *The Immunization Decision: A Guide For Parents.*

233. *Mosby's Medical and Nursing Dictionary* (1983), p. 483.

234. "Hib Vaccine Efficacy Trials Continue: data needed about use in younger children." *Journal of the American Medical Association,* 1989; 261-2015.

235. Ann Winthrop, "Medical Update: Vaccine Breakthrough." *American Baby,* December 1990; p. 12. The Cahners Publishing Company, a division of Reed Publishing, Newton, Massachusetts.

236. "Hib Vaccine Efficacy Trials Continue: data needed about use in younger children." *Journal of the American Medical Association,* 1989; 261-2015.

237. J.B. Milstien, T.P. Gross, J.N. Kuritsky, "Adverse reactions reported following receipt of Haemophilus influenzae type b vaccine: an analysis after one year of marketing." *Pediatrics* 1987; 80:270-274.

238. Vincent I. Ahonkhai, M.D. *et al.* "Influenzae type b conjugate vaccine (meningococcal protein conjugate) (Ped vax HIB tm): clinical evaluation. *Pediatrics, supplement to, part 2, Current Status of Haemophilus Influenzae type b Vaccines,* vol. 85, No. 4. (American Academy of Pediatrics, April 1990), p. 677.

239. M.T. Osterholm, *et al.* "Lack of efficacy of Haemophilus b polysaccharide vaccine in Minnesota." *Journal of the American Medical Association,* 260:1423, (September 9, 1988).

240. Ibid.

241. Eugene D. Shapiro, M.D. and Anne T. Berg, PhD, "Protective Efficacy of Haemophilus influenzae Type b Polysaccharide Vaccine." *Pediatrics, supplement to, part 2, Current Status of Haemophilus Influenzae type b Vaccines,* Vol. 85, No. 4. (American Academy of Pediatrics, April 1990), p. 646.

242. Ibid.

243. Geoffrey A. Weinberg, M.D. and Dan M. Granoff, M.D., "Immunogenicity of Haemophilus influenzae Type b Polysaccharide-Protein Conjugate vaccines in children with conditions associated with impaired antibody responses to Type b Polysaccharide Vaccine." *Pediatrics, supplement to,*

part 2, *Current Status of Haemophilus Influenzae type b Vaccines*, Vol. 85, No. 4. (American Academy of Pediatrics, April 1990), p. 659.

244. Randall Neustaedter, *The Immunization Decision: A Guide For Parents.*

245. Ibid.

246. Ibid.

247. A.M. Arbeter, S.E. Starr, S.A. Plotkin, "Varicella vaccine studies in healthy children and adults. *Pediatrics* 1986; 78(suppl):748-756, as cited by Randall Neustaedter, *The Immunization Decision: A Guide For Parents.*

248. S. Plotkin, "Hell's fire and varicella-vaccine safety. *New England Journal of Medicine* 1988; 318:573-575, as cited by Randall Neustaedter, *The Immunization Decision: A Guide For Parents.*

249. Randall Neustaedter, *The Immunization Decision: A Guide For Parents.*

250. Ibid.

251. P.A. Brunell, "Varicella vaccine — Where are we?" *Pediatrics* 1986; 78 (suppl):721-722, as cited by Randall Neustaedter, *The Immunization Decision: A Guide For Parents.*

252. Randall Neustaedter, *The Immunization Decision: A Guide For Parents.*

253. "Pneumococcal polysaccharide vaccine." *MMWR* 1989; 38:64-76, as cited by Randall Neustaedter, *The Immunization Decision: A Guide For Parents.*

254. Randall Neustaedter, *The Immunization Decision: A Guide For Parents.*

255. Ibid.

256. Committee on Infectious Diseases, American Academy of Pediatrics. Recommendations for using pneumococcal vaccine in children. *Pediatrics* 1985; 75:1153-1158, as cited by Randall Neustaedter, *The Immunization Decision: A Guide For Parents.*

257. Randall Neustaedter, *The Immunization Decision: A Guide For Parents.*

258. Lisa Lovett, D.C., *Immunity, Why Not Keep It?*

259. William T. O'Connor, M.D., *AIDS: The Alarming Reality*, (fourth edition) (The H.I.V.E. Foundation, PO Box 808, Vacaville, CA 95696, 1988).

260. William Campbell Douglass, M.D., *AIDS: The End of Civilization.* (Valet Publishers, Clayton, GA 30525, 1989).

261. Robert S. Mendelsohn, M.D., "AIDS: Linkage to Smallpox Vaccine, AIDS and Tetanus Vaccine." *The People's Doctor Newsletter,* Vol. 11, No. 8.

262. *The Strecker Memorandum* (video) (The Strecker Group, 1216 Wilshire Blvd., Los Angeles, CA 90017).

263. William T. O'Connor, M.D., *AIDS: The Alarming Reality.*

264. Ibid.

265. *The Strecker Memorandum.*

266. William T. O'Connor, M.D., *AIDS: The Alarming Reality.*

267. Robert S. Mendelsohn, M.D., "AIDS Controversies Escalate." *The People's Doctor Newsletter*, Vol. 10, No. 10.

268. William T. O'Connor, M.D., *AIDS: The Alarming Reality.*
269. Robert S. Mendelsohn, M.D., "AIDS Controversies Escalate."
270. Idem. "AIDS: Linkage to Smallpox Vaccine, AIDS and Tetanus Vaccine."
271. William T. O'Connor.
272. Jennifer Hyman, "Children at Risk: the DPT Dilemma."
273. Gene Antonio, *The AIDS Cover-up?* (Ignatius Press, San Francisco, 1986).
274. William T. O'Connor, M.D., *AIDS: The Alarming Reality.*
275. Prem S. Dev, N.D., B.M.S., G.H.M.S., 28 years clinical experience in homeopathic and naturopathic medicine, interview held at his office in Canby, Oregon, 1987.
276. Randall Neustaedter, *The Immunization Decision: A Guide For Parents.*
277. Idem. "Measles and Homeopathic Immunizations." *Mother to Mother, Another View*, April/May 1990.
278. Harris L. Coulter, *DPT: A Shot in the Dark.*
279. Randall Neustaedter, *The Immunization Decision: A Guide For Parents.*
280. Ibid.
281. Lisa Lovett, D.C., *Immunity, Why Not Keep It?*
282. Walene James, *Immunization: The Reality Behind the Myth.*
283. *Whooping Cough, the DPT Vaccine and Reducing Vaccine Reactions.*
284. Walene James, *Immunization: The Reality Behind the Myth.*
285. Randall Neustaedter, *The Immunization Decision: A Guide For Parents.*
286. *How to Legally Avoid Unwanted Immunizations of All Kinds.* (Humanitarian Publishing Company, R.D. 3, Clymer Rd., Quakertown, PA 18951).
287. Walene James, *Immunization: The Reality Behind the Myth.*

ABOUT THE AUTHOR

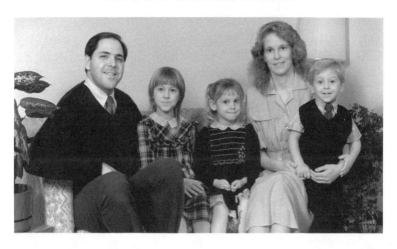

Cynthia Cournoyer is shown here with her husband, Neal Cournoyer and their children, Jennifer, 9, Amanda, 5 and John, 2 ½. Cynthia graduated in 1979 from California State University at Northridge with a Bachelor of Arts degree in Geography. She is also a certified childbirth educator. Cynthia became interested in the vaccine issue shortly after the birth of their first child. She has compiled information on vaccines over the last nine years. *What About Immunizations?* began as a pamphlet she gave to any parent asking questions about vaccines. Many conversations with parents across the nation revealed a need that Cynthia tried to fill with earlier editions of *What About Immunizations?* It finally grew into this fifth edition. She continues to be motivated to research and to refine her perspective on the vaccine philosophy in order to help other parents, like herself, who are searching for the common sense approach to vaccine decision-making.

If you cannot obtain a copy of *What About Immunizations?* locally, send $10.95 to:

D. Nelson
P.O. Box 2302
Santa Cruz, CA 95063

What About Immunizations? is available to anyone at a wholesale discount. For further information, call: 1-800-877-1267

NOTES